Frances T. Giedt, and
Bonnie S. Polin, Ph.D.,
with the Nutritional Services Staff
at Joslin Diabetes Center

Other Books by These Authors
The Joslin Diabetes Gourmet Cookbook

The Joslin Diabetes

Quick and Easy Cookbook

{ 200 Recipes for }
{ 1 to 4 People }

A Fireside Book

Published by Simon & Schuster

FIRESIDE
Rockefeller Center
1230 Avenue of the Americas
New York, NY 10020

DESIGNED BY RALPH FOWLER

Manufactured in the United States of America

3   5   7   9   10   8   6   4

Library of Congress Cataloging-in-Publication Data

Giedt, Frances Towner.
The Joslin diabetes quick and easy cookbook : 200 recipes for 1 to 4 people / Frances T. Giedt
and Bonnie S. Polin with the nutritional services staff at Joslin Diabetes Center.
p.   cm.
Includes index.
1. Diabetes—Diet therapy—Recipes.   I. Polin, Bonnie Sanders, 1941–   .   II. Joslin Diabetes Center.
III. Title.
RC662.G54   1998
641.5'6314—dc21   98-27498
CIP

ISBN 0-684-83923-7

Contents

Breakfast   23

Power Lunches   66

Foreword

When food tastes good, eating is one of the most pleasurable activities in which we can partake. When food is not only delicious but also healthy and prepared especially for the diabetes patient and the patient's family, then eating can be a true delight. As the Medical Director of the Joslin Diabetes Center and a clinician who has worked with diabetes patients and their families for the past eighteen years, it is a real pleasure to write the foreword for this remarkable culinary resource. ❡ Many cookbooks are available that include low-fat and low-sugar recipes. These vary considerably in one important area: how good the food tastes. This book is unique because it combines a wealth of information resulting from a team effort by Frances Giedt and Bonnie Polin, Ph.D., along with the Nutrition Department at the Joslin Diabetes Center. They created excellent recipes satisfying the needs of diabetes patients as well as the dietary needs and desires of family members. The book makes it easy to prepare many tasty meals, appetizers, desserts, and snacks to serve family and friends, and it also provides information about the "story behind the story" in cooking to maximize health. This combination makes the book a terrific resource not only for diabetic patients but for all who want an approach to healthy eating.

There is now considerable agreement about what constitutes a healthy diet. Experts representing the American Diabetes Association, American Heart Association, and other societies have reached consensus that it is important in general to decrease the amount of saturated fats in our diets, eat more complex carbohydrates and fiber than are typically consumed by Americans, and consume adequate but not excessive amounts of protein. The food charts that many of us have grown up with have been tilted in a new direction, one that emphasizes grains, fruits, and vegetables, rather than traditional meat, potato, and dairy foods. This book provides delicious ways to translate that nutritional expertise into fun eating. It is also great for people who want to eat in a more healthy fashion to prevent diabetes, lose weight, and decrease the risk of high blood pressure, heart disease, and cancer, and, in general, cut down on obesity and related disorders.

We at Joslin have had a long-standing tradition of putting the patient and the family in charge of their health. This has led us to place a heavy emphasis on teaching people about diabetes and its care, and how they can increase their knowledge of diabetes. Since diet is one of the key aspects of the proper care for diabetes, this book becomes part of that learning—a teaching that is also a rewarding experience of cooking meals for the family. (Questions that come up in the course of reading and using the cookbook should always be addressed to members of your health care team including your physician, dietitian, and nurse educator.) The combination of healthy eating and an active lifestyle that includes walking, hiking, biking, and other exercise is a wonderful way for families to have fun and enjoyment together.

Alan M. Jacobson, M.D.
Medical Director
Joslin Diabetes Center

Introductions

This book is dedicated to those people with diabetes who cook for themselves and those who cook for diabetics. They may have a hundred things on their schedule but still want to prepare a healthy meal that not only looks and tastes interesting and delicious but also conforms to the needs of someone with diabetes for wholesome food prepared with a minimum of fat and controlled amounts of protein and sodium. ¶ As diabetics ourselves, we understand the dilemma since we do not always have time to spend in the kitchen; yet good, nutritious food is a priority in our lives. The recipes in this book reflect the way we cook and eat every day.

Some special thoughts: It has now been almost ten years since I was diagnosed as having type 2 diabetes. Looking back on that day and reflecting on the changes in my life, I see how food is integrally tied to our emotions, our lifestyles, and our family and cultural values. As the author of nine cookbooks, I have devoted my career to developing and testing recipes, and can see the direct effects of food on the management of my disease. I have learned firsthand that a high level of fat (particularly saturated fat) can cause long-term complications for the person with diabetes. Not only does fat contribute to weight gain, making control of blood sugar levels even more difficult—causing small blood vessel diseases that affect the eyes, kidneys, and nervous system—but at high levels certain fats can also lead to problems related to large blood vessel diseases, causing angina (chest pain), heart attack, stroke, and poor blood circulation.

When I've taught cooking classes for people with diabetes and lectured at hospitals and clinics, I've been amazed at the number of people with diabetes who don't recognize the seriousness of the disease until complications set in. And as I chat with other people with diabetes on the Internet, I realize that food is the center of their world. Everyone seems to be desperately searching for the "magic diet" that will help them control their blood sugars. To say that people with diabetes are "foodies" is no exaggeration. Many are well armed with nutritional information gleaned from the airwaves, bookstores, and newsstands. And while they sometimes know what they should be eating, they choose to eat improper food because their "diabetic" food was frequently lacking one critical ingredient—taste. When fat, sugar, and salt (three important transmitters of flavor) are removed from food, the result is often bland and boring. If food doesn't taste wonderful, no one wants to eat it—no matter how healthy it is or how well it controls blood sugar and blood fat levels.

This is why I am particularly pleased to be once again teamed with my co-author, Bonnie Polin, and the registered dietitians, diabetes educators, and doctors at the world-renowned Joslin Diabetes Center to create another cookbook for people with diabetes. In our earlier collaboration (*The Joslin Diabetes Gourmet Cookbook*), we developed hundreds of delicious good-for-you recipes, but many of the dishes required one to spend a fair amount of time in the kitchen. As our lives get busier, we're faced with the dilemma: It's usually easy to prepare a delicious, healthy meal on a weekend, but during the rest of the week, who has time to cook?

Fret no longer. We've developed more than two hundred mouth-watering low-fat recipes that you can cook in under thirty minutes. These recipes are full of vibrant flavor, eye-catching color, pleasing texture, and, most important, a healthful balance of nutrients. Using this book will help you rethink the vast number of food choices now available to you—without compromising your health for good taste.

Since many of us, Bonnie and myself included, are no longer cooking for a large family, we designed the majority of the recipes for two servings. Should you want or need to cook for more than two, the recipes can easily be doubled or tripled (we've noted any that might need modifications).

These are recipes for you to cook and enjoy forever. They're simple, delicious, and quick. More important, the recipes will help you make changes in your diet that will result in better control of your diabetes. So let's start cooking.

Frances Towner Giedt
Arlington, Texas

When I think about living with diabetes, I recall an image of twenty years ago—my friend's grandmother, a Southern lady of around seventy, floating down a spiral staircase in a ball gown, making a grand entrance. She is well into her nineties now and has had diabetes for many decades; she also remains the beloved matriarch of her family. She never stopped taking care of herself or others. Years later, when I developed type 1 diabetes, the memory of this elegant and emotionally strong woman gave me hope that I, too, could take care of myself and still live a full and rewarding life.

I have been instrumental in helping others and myself by developing and conducting a diabetes clinic for the working poor. In this clinic a very popular exercise has been to get a person to list everything in his or her refrigerator and freezer, and then come up with a series of quick and easy meals that are delicious and healthy at the same time. This exercise came about because patients complained that healthy cooking was too difficult. The results of the exercise were always a real surprise for the group because we improvised mouthwatering recipes like Three-Pepper Mexican Pizza and Breakfast Banana Splits. These people who had once been turned off to healthy eating were suddenly turned on. It was an incredibly rewarding experience for me because for the first time people expressed hope. They said they would try—a major step, since many had been referred by their health team because of "noncompliance."

Many people feel trapped by their diabetes; they eat bland food while their family members continue to eat the way they always have. In our sessions they learned it was possible to prepare low-fat, low-protein meals to be enjoyed by the family and not just the person with diabetes. Variations on the recipes ranged from all-American to Asian foods as well, depending on the group, but they were always inspiring.

The idea for this book grew out of the desire by many diabetics for a compilation of quick and easy recipes that are familiar to all of us. The recipes therefore consist of what we have always liked to eat. The idea of comfort food is not new but is important to those who feel deprived by their disease. We are pleased to offer you delicious recipes that you and others will enjoy; you'd hardly suspect that they are also good for you.

Forget the old saying "Too many cooks spoil the broth." My coauthor, Frances Giedt, made this collaboration a pleasure. In addition, our colleagues at Joslin offered wonderful feedback and their expertise. The result, I hope, will assist you in taking hold of your life in a positive and healthy way—similar to that Southern lady whose grace, fortitude, and lifestyle qualified her as a role model for us all. I wish you a long life filled with good health. *Bon appétit.*

Bonnie Sanders Polin, Ph.D.
Tulsa, Oklahoma

About Joslin Diabetes Center

Joslin Diabetes Center, affiliated with Harvard Medical School, is preeminent in diabetes research and treatment in the nation and indeed in the world. As such, it is fitting that Joslin published the definitive guide to diabetes self-care, *The Joslin Guide to Diabetes: A Program for Managing Your Treatment* (a Fireside Book published by Simon & Schuster in 1995), by Richard S. Beaser, M.D., with Joan V. C. Hill, R.D., C.D.E. It is an indispensable resource for everybody with the disease. ❡ The oldest free-standing institution in the United States dedicated solely to diabetes research, patient care, and patient and professional education, Joslin Diabetes Center was founded in 1898 in Boston by Elliott P. Joslin, M.D., a pioneer in the field of diabetes who believed that the patient was an integral part of the diabetes treatment team.

The Joslin facility takes up an entire city block in Boston's famous Longwood Medical Area of Harvard-affiliated hospitals and institutions. Its outstanding staff—including endocrinologists, ophthalmologists, renal specialists, exercise physiologists, podiatrists, psychiatrists, psychologists, social workers, nurses, dietitians, certified diabetes educators, and others—has provided total quality care every day to hundreds of thousands of patients. Joslin's cadre of scientists conduct basic and clinical research that is immediately translated into new and better ways to treat people with diabetes. One major development was the invention of laser surgery for diabetic retinopathy.

Since 1987, Joslin Diabetes Center has established affiliated treatment centers throughout the country and is working directly with hospitals around the world. You will find listings for the Joslin Diabetes Center and its affiliates in Appendix Four.

A Note from the Joslin Diabetes Center

As Director of Educational Services and Programs at the Joslin Diabetes Center, I have come to realize that education about diabetes does not come overnight. Not only that, but I have also come to realize that just because you are educated doesn't mean you don't struggle with how to take better care of yourself. Working with the team to bring this book together, Fran, Bonnie, Jill, and the dietitians at Joslin have raised my awareness of two barriers to better control: poor self-esteem and the need to punish. ❡ It does not make sense to punish yourself for what you aren't able to do. The daily "chores" required to live well with diabetes are complex. Learning to problem-solve, to set goals, and to determine ways to accomplish those goals is a challenge. With your team—family, educators, and doctors—to help in your journey, you can achieve success.

I am pleased to carry on the tradition of Elliott Joslin's philosophy with the help of Julie Rafferty in the communications department and our dear friend, the late Ray Moloney. Without their expertise, this new book would not be available to help you put theory into practice.

Joan Hill, R.D., C.D.E.
Director of Educational Services and Programs
Joslin Diabetes Center

Karen Chalmers, M.S., R.D., CDE., Director of Nutrition

Nutrition and Diabetes Educators:
Lisa Casey, R.D., C.N.S.D., C.D.E.
Emmy Friedlander, M.S., R.D., C.D.E.
Kevin Harrington, R.D.
Roberta Laredo, R.D., C.D.E.
Melinda Maryniuk, M.Ed., R.D., C.D.E., F.A.D.A.
Lois Maurer, M.S., R.D., C.D.E.
Amy Peterson, M.S., R.D., C.D.E.

Guidelines for Living with Diabetes
"Strive for a Healthier You"

- Eat a variety of foods, guided by your individualized meal plan.

- Avoid foods high in fat (daily intake should not exceed 30 percent calories from fat), saturated fat (no more than 10 percent calories from saturated fat), and cholesterol (a limit of 300 milligrams per day).

- At least half of your food intake should come from vegetables, fruits, and grain products.

- Use sugar in moderation.

- Use salt and high-sodium products in moderation.

- Check with your health care team on the use of alcoholic beverages; if approved, use in moderation.

- Drink six to eight glasses of water a day, not including the fluids contained in coffee, tea, and diet beverages.

- Strive to obtain and maintain a healthy weight.

- Exercise daily to help with losing weight and staying fit.

- Seek ways to minimize stress.

- Learn everything you can about food and how it affects your blood sugar levels with self-monitoring of blood glucose.

- Do not view having to take medication as being a failure; view it as a way to achieve better control of your blood sugar and blood fat levels.

- Problem-solve with your health care team about taking care of your diabetes on special occasions such as travel, sick days, and so forth, so that you can feel in control.

A Healthy Short-Order Pantry

Cooking for yourself if you're diabetic or for someone with diabetes is a day-to-day lifetime commitment to healthy cooking. Since this book is geared to those who cook for one or two people most of the time, your pantry is likely to look quite different from that of a family with young children and other family members dropping in for meals. ❡ Buying for two need not be difficult. The goal is to avoid waste and leftovers, so you must think small. Stock your pantry and refrigerator with small amounts of the best you can afford and keep the inventory turning. Spices lose their flavor with age, and oil loses its freshness. Learn to select small basic vegetables, such as onions, carrots, and potatoes.

Reevaluate your kitchen storage. How and where you store foods can make a difference. We keep spices in view so they're handy to use, but away from the stove because they fare better when kept cool and dry. Beans, grains, and pastas are stored in clear jars. Garlic and shallots are stored in a special ceramic jar. Onions, potatoes, and winter squashes are kept in baskets. Citrus and other fruits sit in a fruit bowl so we'll remember to use them.

Many of our recipes call for fat-free reduced-sodium broth. If there is any left after making the dish, pour the remainder into airtight freezer storage bags in ¼-cup portions, arrange on a baking sheet, and freeze until firm. Store in the freezer to use as needed.

Here are the items we keep on hand for quick, healthy cooking:

Vinegars

Balsamic: Italian, sweet, and dark; used sparingly on salads, fresh fruits, in marinades, and as a sauce for vegetables, meats, and poultry

Fruit-infused: with no sugar added; raspberry and blueberry are excellent on salads and vegetables as well as for a base for sauces

Herb-infused: with basil, tarragon, fruit peels, chiles, garlic, or shallots. Use for salads and sauces

Red wine: excellent on salads

White wine: good on chicken, potato, and vegetable salads

Sherry wine: fuller and less acidic than other wine vinegars; wonderful on salads and excellent in seafood and chicken dishes

Other vinegars worth having are champagne, cider, malt, and rice wine.

Cooking Sprays

Cooking sprays are useful because they have no calories and yet stop foods from sticking, aid in their cooking, and add flavor. Purchase olive oil, butter-flavored,

A Guide to Healthy Oils

All oils have approximately 14 grams of fat and 120 calories per tablespoon. Where they differ is in taste and the percentage of saturated fats; these cause the body to produce more cholesterol. Oils that you'll need for our recipes are marked with an asterisk. Others are nice to have for variety of flavor. Remember that all oils are 100 percent fat and should be used sparingly.

	POLYUNSATURATED (%)	MONOUNSATURATED (%)	SATURATED (%)
Almond	18	73	8
Avocado	13	71	4
Canola*	30	59	7
Corn	59	24	13
Grapeseed	69	0	10
Hazelnut	10	78	7
Olive*	8	74	13
Peanut	32	46	17
Safflower	13	9	0
Sesame*	42	40	14
Sunflower	68	21	11
Vegetable	74	12	9
Walnut	67	24	9

and vegetable cooking sprays. Do try various brands because they have different tastes, and you'll want to find the ones you consider most pleasing.

Grains

Quick-cooking rice: white, brown, basmati
Quick-cooking couscous
Kasha
Quick-cooking oats (rolled oats)

Instant polenta
Instant potato flakes
Stone-ground cornmeal: white and yellow

Legumes

Canned black beans, cannelini, garbanzo (chick peas), navy, and white beans

Black-eyed peas
Lentils: red and brown

Pasta

Angel hair
Bow ties (farfalle)
Linguine
Oriental rice stick noodles

Penne
Quick-cooking lasagna
Rotini
Spaghetti

Baking Needs

Unbleached flour
Nonfat pancake mix
Graham cracker crumbs
Cornstarch
Dry bread crumbs (unseasoned)
Baking powder
Baking soda
Cream of tartar

Cocoa powder
Salt and kosher salt
Vanilla extract
Artificial sweetener
Sugar
Honey
Brown sugar

Canned and Packaged Goods

No-salt-added tomato paste

No-salt-added canned tomatoes

Fat-free reduced-sodium broth: beef, chicken, and vegetable

Reduced-sodium soy sauce

Canned pumpkin

Reduced-sodium ketchup

No-sugar-added fruit spread

Natural peanut butter

No-sugar-added dried fruit: cherries, apples, apricots, peaches, currants, golden raisins

Evaporated skim milk

Powdered buttermilk

Worcestershire sauce

Hot pepper sauce

Mustard: Dijon, regular, coarse-grain

Unsweetened fruit juices

Dry red and dry white wine for cooking

Cognac for cooking

Dry sherry for cooking

Tequila for cooking

Spices

Ground allspice

Dill: seed and weed

Caraway seed

Celery flakes

Celery seed

Chili powder

Ground cinnamon

Cloves: ground and whole

Coriander: ground and seeds

Ground cumin

Curry powder: mild and imported Indian

Fennel seed

Ground ginger

Paprika

Poppy seed

Crushed red pepper flakes

Vegetable flakes

In the Freezer

Frozen fruit and berries—no sugar added

Concentrated frozen fruit juices

Puff pastry dough

Pastry dough

Reduced-calorie margarine

Boneless, skinless chicken breasts, pounded and individually wrapped

Ground white turkey breast in ½-pound packages

Extra-lean ground beef sirloin (10 percent fat) in ½-pound packages or individual 2-ounce patties

Turkey cutlets, individually wrapped

Nuts

Vegetables in bags: corn,
chopped green bell peppers,
chopped onions, peas, potatoes, spinach, and so forth

Breads and rolls: sliced whole
wheat, multigrain, fat-free
French, pita

In the Refrigerator

Part-skim Parmesan cheese
Fat-free mozzarella cheese
Part-skim mozzarella cheese
Fat-free ricotta cheese
Fat-free cream cheese
Reduced-fat margarine
Fat-free sour cream
Fresh ginger
Lemons
Oranges
Fresh fruit in season
Fresh fruit juices
Scallions

Fresh herbs and parsley
Plain nonfat yogurt
Salad ingredients: lettuces,
bell peppers, celery, carrots,
cucumbers, radishes, and
so forth
Fresh vegetables in season
Dill pickles (if your diet allows
them)
Tomato paste in a tube
Egg substitute
Eggs
Skim milk

Miscellaneous

Garlic
Onions

Potatoes: red and russet
Shallots

Reading Food Labels

Thanks to the new federal food label regulations, everyone can obtain a complete list of ingredients, standard serving sizes, and reliable health and content claims in a reader-friendly format. You can now make informed food choices by reading the food label. ❡ The first item to check is the serving size. It is the basis for the nutritional information and may be less or more than you would normally eat, so you will need to account for the difference. ❡ The label states the calorie content per serving of the product and how many of the calories come from fat. It must list the amount of saturated fat, cholesterol, sodium, total carbohydrates (dietary fiber and sugar), and protein. You'll also find the content for vitamins A and C as well as calcium and iron.

In addition, the label must also display daily values, a percentage based on a 2,000-calorie daily diet. Your daily values may be higher or lower depending on your calorie intake.

Many label terms now have definitions set by the Food and Drug Administration. Here are some of the common terms you'll find on the front labels of food packages:

Fat-free: has less than 0.5 gram of fat per serving

Cholesterol-free: 2 or fewer milligrams of cholesterol per serving

Sodium-free: fewer than 5 milligrams of sodium per serving

Calorie-free: fewer than 5 calories per serving

Low-fat: 3 grams or less of fat per serving

Low saturated fat: less than 1 gram of saturated fat per serving

Low-sodium: less than 140 milligrams of sodium per serving

Very low sodium: less than 35 milligrams of sodium per serving

Nutrition Facts

Serving Size ½ cup (114 g)
Servings Per Container 4

Amount Per Serving

Calories 260   Calories From Fat 120

	% Daily Value*
Total Fat 13 g	20%
Saturated Fat 5 g	25%
Cholesterol 30 mg	10%
Sodium 660 mg	28%
Total Carbohydrate 31 g	10%
Dietary Fiber 0 g	0%
Sugars 5 g	
Protein 5 g	

Vitamin A 4%	•	Vitamin C 2%
Calcium 15%	•	Iron 4%

*Percent Daily Values are based on a 2,000 calorie diet. Your daily values may be higher or lower depending on your calorie needs:

	Calories:	2,000	2,500
Total Fat	Less than	65 g	80 g
Sat Fat	Less than	20 g	25 g
Cholesterol	Less than	300 mg	300 mg
Sodium	Less than	2,400 mg	2,400 mg
Total Carbohydrate		300 g	375 g
Dietary Fiber		25 g	30 g

Calories per gram:
Fat 9   •   Carbohydrate 4   •   Protein 4

Low-cholesterol: less than 20 milligrams of cholesterol per serving

Low-calorie: 40 calories or less per serving

Reduced: the product has been nutritionally altered and now contains 25 percent less of a given nutrient or 25 percent fewer calories than the regular product

Nutrition Information

Our recipes contain nutrition and diabetes exchange information calculated by Jill West, R.D., C.D.E., a nutrition and diabetes consultant in Davis, California, using the most current data available from ESHA Research *The Food Processor* (Version 2.2), the United States Department of Agriculture, and from manufacturer food label information when necessary.

Percentage of Calories from Fat

The recommended daily guideline is 30 percent of calories from fat. An entire day's meal plan should not derive more than 30 percent of the total calories from fat—*not* of the calories per recipe or per meal. The percentage of calories from fat listed in each recipe is a guideline: If a recipe contains a relatively high percentage of fat, the rest of that meal and that day's other meals should compensate for the rich dish. Be sure to check the total calories and total fat grams, because sometimes a recipe is so low in calories that the fat percentage looks exorbitant but in fact is just a gram or two. The total grams of fat are important. On a 2,000-calorie daily allowance, for instance, you want to keep your total fat grams to less than 67 and your total saturated fat grams to less than 20.

BREAKFAST

{ Eggs and Meats }

Mushroom Omelet

This omelet calls for cultivated white button mushrooms, but if you happen to have fresh wild mushrooms on hand, by all means use them. Stay clear of canned or jarred mushrooms, because they're high in sodium. Use frozen mushrooms if fresh aren't available.

> *butter-flavored cooking spray*
> *6 ounces mixed mushrooms, such as portobello, button, shiitake, cremini, thinly sliced*
> *2 scallions (white part plus 1 inch of green), thinly sliced*
> *1 cup egg substitute*
> *1 ounce fat-free cream cheese, cut into ¼-inch dice*
> *freshly ground pepper to taste*
> *1 teaspoon minced fresh thyme leaves or ¼ teaspoon crushed dried*

Lightly coat a nonstick 8- or 9-inch sauté pan with cooking spray. Add the mushrooms and scallions and cook over medium-high heat, stirring occasionally, until soft and all liquid has evaporated, about 5 minutes. Be careful not to let the scallions burn.

Add the egg substitute and diced cheese. Lower the heat to medium and cook without stirring until the omelet starts to bubble around the edges, about 10 seconds. Then stir, pushing the mixture toward the center of the pan.

When the bottom is set but the top is still slightly wet and creamy, carefully slide the omelet out of the pan onto a serving platter. Flip one half over the other half to form a half-circle. Cut the omelet in half. Serve immediately.

Makes 2 servings.

PER SERVING: 99 calories (4% calories from fat), <1 g total fat (trace saturated fat), 16 g protein, 8 g carbohydrates, 1 g dietary fiber, 1 mg cholesterol, 273 mg sodium

JOSLIN EXCHANGES: 2 very low fat protein, 1 vegetable

Note: If doubling this recipe, make two small omelets rather than one larger one, because they are easier to control.

Asian Omelet with Crab

This Chinese-style dish is reminiscent of egg foo yung but lacks the fat and salt of that classic dish. You'll never miss them as you enjoy the mélange of tastes.

1 cup egg substitute
4 ounces fresh crab meat, picked over, or imitation crab meat
1 cup fresh mung bean sprouts
1 scallion (white part plus 1 inch of green), thinly sliced
1 clove garlic, minced, or ⅛ teaspoon garlic powder
½ teaspoon minced fresh ginger or to taste
½ teaspoon canola oil

In a medium bowl, combine egg substitute, crab meat, bean sprouts, scallion, garlic, and ginger.

Heat a small nonstick skillet and add half of the oil. (This little bit of oil helps crisp the eggs.) Pour in half of the egg mixture and cook over medium-high heat until brown on the bottom. Turn and cook until brown on the other side. Transfer the omelet to a serving plate and keep warm. Repeat the process, using the remaining oil and egg mixture. Serve immediately.

Makes 2 servings.

PER SERVING: 142 calories (14% calories from fat), 2 g total fat (0.2 g saturated fat), 24 g protein, 6 g carbohydrates, 1 g dietary fiber, 30 mg cholesterol, 811 mg sodium

JOSLIN EXCHANGES: 3 very low fat protein, 1 vegetable

Tomato Frittata

A frittata—an Italian omelet filled with potatoes, onions, and vegetables—finishes cooking in a hot oven to make it a bit drier than a regular omelet. It is not fussy about its timing, making it one of our favorites for brunch, lunch, or supper. These omelets can be served piping hot right from the oven or allowed to cool to room temperature—perfect for the picnic basket.

olive oil cooking spray
1 scallion (white part plus 2 inches of green), thinly sliced
1 cup egg substitute
2 medium plum tomatoes, thinly sliced
½ cup (2 ounces) shredded fat-free mozzarella cheese
1 tablespoon grated Parmesan cheese
4 small fresh basil leaves or 1 teaspoon crushed dried
⅛ teaspoon dried garlic powder (optional)
freshly ground pepper to taste

Preheat the broiler. Lightly coat a 9-inch ovenproof nonstick sauté pan with the cooking spray. Add the scallion and sauté over medium heat for 1 minute, until wilted. Add the egg substitute and turn the heat to medium-low. Arrange the tomato slices in overlapping layers on top of the egg. Cover with the mozzarella and Parmesan cheeses. Sprinkle with the basil, garlic, and pepper.

Cook until the bottom is just set and the top is still wet, 4 to 5 minutes. Place the pan under the broiler until the top is puffed, sizzling, and set, 1 to 2 minutes. Remove from the broiler and, using a plastic spatula, slide the frittata onto a serving platter. Cut into 4 wedges.

Makes 2 servings.

PER SERVING: 126 calories (9% calories from fat), 1 g total fat (0.6 g saturated fat), 21 g protein, 8 g carbohydrates, 1 g dietary fiber, 3 mg cholesterol, 541 mg sodium

JOSLIN EXCHANGES: 3 very low fat protein, 1 vegetable

Garden Frittata

This golden pancake-style omelet will be a main-course brunch favorite. You can be as creative as you wish with regard to the vegetables, varying them according to season, preference, or what's on hand in the fridge.

olive oil cooking spray
1 small new potato, chopped into ¼-inch dice
4 ounces thin asparagus, woody ends snapped off, cut into 2-inch pieces
2 cups lightly packed torn small spinach leaves, washed and dried
1 cup egg substitute
1½ teaspoons minced fresh thyme or ½ teaspoon crushed dried
¼ cup shredded fat-free mozzarella cheese
¼ cup diced red bell pepper
freshly ground pepper to taste
chopped fresh parsley for garnish (optional)

Preheat the broiler. Lightly coat a 9-inch ovenproof nonstick sauté pan with cooking spray.

Add the diced potato and cook over medium-high heat, turning frequently, for 5 to 8 minutes, until easily pierced with the tip of a sharp knife. Add the asparagus and cook, stir-frying for 2 to 3 minutes, until the asparagus is barely tender. Add the spinach and stir-fry for another minute, until the spinach wilts.

Turn the heat to medium and pour in the egg substitute. Sprinkle with the thyme, cheese, diced red pepper, and pepper. Cook, stirring lightly, until the frittata begins to set, about 5 minutes.

Place the frittata under the broiler until it puffs and is golden brown, 2 to 3 minutes. Using a plastic spatula, slide the frittata onto a serving plate and cut into 4 wedges. Sprinkle with parsley and serve immediately or cool to room temperature.

Makes 2 servings.

PER SERVING: 143 calories (2% calories from fat), <1 g total fat (trace saturated fat), 18 g protein, 18 g carbohydrates, 2 g dietary fiber, trace cholesterol, 342 mg sodium

JOSLIN EXCHANGES: 2 very low fat protein, 1 carbohydrate (1 bread/starch), 1 vegetable

Huevos Rancheros

Eggs need not be totally shunned by people with diabetes. To reduce the risk of cardiovascular disease, one should limit cholesterol intake to less than 300 milligrams per day. Since a large egg has 213 milligrams of cholesterol, you'll need to watch your other high-cholesterol foods for the rest of that day. ❡ But when it comes to a quick, soul-satisfying, and inexpensive brunch dish, this one is hard to beat. It's recommended that you should have no more than two or three eggs per week.

1 recipe Fresh Tomato Salsa (page 97)
2 tablespoons water
½ teaspoon crushed dried oregano
2 large eggs
salt (optional)
freshly ground pepper to taste
1 cup canned black beans, drained and rinsed
½ tablespoon white wine vinegar
3 to 5 dashes hot pepper sauce or to taste
2 6-inch corn tortillas
2 tablespoons reduced-fat sharp cheddar cheese
chopped cilantro for garnish (optional)

Preheat the broiler.

Place the salsa, water, and oregano in a medium-heavy skillet. Heat over medium-low heat until the mixture starts to bubble. Crack the eggs one at a time into the liquid without breaking the yolks. Sprinkle with salt (if using) and pepper to taste. Poach the eggs, keeping the liquid just below boiling to avoid breaking the egg whites, until the eggs are cooked to desired doneness, 3 to 5 minutes.

Meanwhile, in a small saucepan, heat the beans, vinegar, and hot pepper sauce. Soften the tortillas by heating them directly on a stovetop burner over medium heat for about 30 seconds, turning frequently. Place them side by side on a heat-proof dish. Spoon half of the bean mixture over each tortilla.

Carefully spoon a poached egg and some of the salsa onto each tortilla and top with the cheese. Broil, 4 to 6 inches from source of heat, until the cheese melts, about 1 minute. Garnish with chopped cilantro if desired. Serve immediately.

Makes 2 servings.

PER SERVING: 274 calories (26% calories from fat), 8 g total fat (2.5 g saturated fat), 18 g protein, 34 g carbohydrates, 8 g dietary fiber, 218 mg cholesterol, 538 mg sodium

JOSLIN EXCHANGES: 2 low-fat protein, 2 carbohydrate (2 bread/starch), 1 vegetable

Brunch Tomato Strata

Make-ahead dishes like this delicious strata are ideal for a lazy morning brunch. Assemble the casseroles the night before to pop in the oven and bake as you're getting dressed for the day. ❧ Whether headed out for a new exhibit at a museum, a brisk walk in the park or mall, or a few links at the golf course, you'll find this savory strata will fortify you for an active day—and it's also ideal for a light supper. ❧ You'll need two 2-cup (16-ounce) oval or round individual casseroles to make this recipe.

olive oil cooking spray
¼ cup frozen chopped onion
¼ cup chopped red bell pepper
1 clove garlic, minced
2 cups cubed Italian bread (about 4 slices)
1 large ripe tomato, cored and sliced crosswise into 6 slices
¼ cup (1 ounce) shredded reduced-fat extra-sharp cheddar cheese
1 tablespoon grated Parmesan cheese
¾ cup evaporated skim milk
½ cup egg substitute
¼ teaspoon crushed dried Italian seasoning
⅛ teaspoon dry mustard
⅛ teaspoon freshly ground pepper
⅛ teaspoon cayenne pepper

Lightly coat a nonstick skillet with cooking spray. Add the onion, bell pepper, and garlic. Sauté over medium-low heat until the onion wilts, about 4 minutes. Remove from the heat.

Lightly coat two 2-cup oval or round individual casseroles with cooking spray. Mix together the bread cubes and onion mixture. Spoon into the casseroles, dividing equally. Arrange 3 tomato slices on top of each casserole. Sprinkle evenly with the 2 cheeses.

In a medium bowl, whisk together the evaporated milk, egg substitute, Italian seasoning, dry mustard, pepper, and cayenne pepper. Pour over the tomato-bread mixture. Cover with foil and chill in the refrigerator overnight or for at least 8 hours.

Preheat the oven to 350°F. Bake the strata, uncovered, for 25 to 30 minutes, until a knife inserted in the center comes out clean. Let stand for 5 minutes before serving.

Makes 2 servings.

PER SERVING: 361 calories (16% calories from fat), 6 g total fat (3 g saturated fat), 26 g protein, 50 g carbohydrates, 4 g dietary fiber, 16 mg cholesterol, 741 mg sodium

JOSLIN EXCHANGES: 1½ low-fat protein, 3 carbohydrate (1 skim milk, 2 bread/starch), 1 vegetable

Open-Faced Breakfast Sandwich

We love eggs Benedict, so we've devised an open-faced sandwich that is equally as flavorful and soul-satisfying, and modified to meet our nutritional goals. Serve this for a leisurely Sunday brunch or light supper. ❡ We prefer the flavor of shiitake mushrooms in this dish, but you can substitute cultivated fresh button mushrooms.

butter-flavored cooking spray
1 medium onion, thinly sliced and separated into rings
¼ pound fresh shiitake mushrooms, thinly sliced
1 tablespoon minced fresh ginger
2 tablespoons fat-free reduced-sodium canned chicken broth
salt (optional)
freshly ground pepper to taste
2 large eggs
2 crumpets or 1 English muffin, split
chopped fresh chervil or flat-leaf parsley for garnish (optional)

Lightly coat a heavy skillet with cooking spray. Add the onion and cook over low heat, stirring often, until the onion is soft and golden, about 4 minutes. Add the mushrooms, ginger, and broth. Cover and continue to cook until the mushrooms are tender and the liquid is absorbed, about 5 minutes. Season with salt (if using) and pepper to taste.

Meanwhile, poach the eggs in simmering water to desired doneness. Toast the crumpets or English muffin.

To serve, place 1 crumpet or ½ English muffin on each of 2 serving plates. Top each crumpet or muffin half with half of the onion-mushroom mixture. Using a slotted spoon, carefully remove the eggs from the poaching liquid and place in the center of each serving. If desired, garnish with chopped chervil. Serve immediately.

Makes 2 servings.

PER SERVING: 208 calories (25% calories from fat), 6 g total fat (1.7 g saturated fat), 10 g protein, 30 g carbohydrates, 4 g dietary fiber, 214 mg cholesterol, 207 mg sodium

JOSLIN EXCHANGES: 1 medium-fat protein, 1 carbohydrate (1 bread/starch), 2 vegetable

Breakfast Burrito

This dish comes together in less than 10 minutes, making it perfect for mornings when you're running late. Wrapped in a napkin or paper towel, it becomes a portable food that can be eaten out of hand while waiting for the bus or train.

butter-flavored cooking spray
¼ cup frozen chopped onion
1 tablespoon chopped canned green chiles, drained
1 cup egg substitute
2 tablespoons shredded fat-free Monterey Jack cheese
⅛ teaspoon freshly ground pepper
⅛ teaspoon hot pepper sauce (optional)
2 10-inch 98 percent fat-free flour tortillas, warmed

Lightly coat a 10-inch nonstick skillet with cooking spray. Cook the onion and chiles in the skillet over medium heat for 3 minutes, stirring occasionally. In a small bowl, mix together the egg substitute, cheese, pepper, and hot pepper sauce (if using). Pour into the skillet.

When the mixture begins to set on the bottom, gently lift the cooked portions with a spatula so the uncooked portion can flow to the bottom. Tilt the skillet if necessary. Cook for 3 to 4 minutes, or until the eggs are scrambled to taste but still moist.

Divide the egg mixture between the tortillas, placing it on one-third of each tortilla. Fold up 1 or 2 inches of the lower edge of each tortilla, then roll from the side with the egg on it to form a burrito. Eat immediately.

Makes 2 servings.

PER SERVING: 150 calories (3% calories from fat), 1 g total fat (trace saturated fat), 16 g protein, 22 g carbohydrates, 4 g dietary fiber, 1 mg cholesterol, 262 mg sodium

JOSLIN EXCHANGES: 2 very low fat protein, 1 carbohydrate (1 bread/starch), 1 vegetable

Crustless Spinach Quiche

Make this the day ahead and serve it warm or at room temperature. We prefer to use the occasional egg in this recipe for better texture, but if you want to further cut fat and cholesterol, you can use 6 tablespoons of egg substitute in place of the whole egg and egg white. This will result in 9 calories, 1 gram of fat (0.5 saturated), and 106 milligrams of cholesterol per serving. The exchanges will not be affected. ❡ This recipe is really best made with fresh spinach. (If you use frozen spinach, be sure to squeeze it very dry.) Happily, most supermarkets sell prewashed fresh spinach in bags. Nevertheless, give the leaves a quick spritz at the sink and then quickly drain them on paper towels.

> *olive oil cooking spray*
> *⅓ cup frozen chopped onion*
> *4 button mushrooms, sliced*
> *1 large plum tomato, chopped*
> *1 cup loosely packed chopped fresh spinach leaves*
> *1 whole large egg plus 1 egg white*
> *½ cup 1% low-fat milk*
> *½ teaspoon Dijon mustard*
> *1 teaspoon chopped parsley*
> *1 teaspoon chopped fresh tarragon or ¼ teaspoon crushed dried*
> *¼ teaspoon salt (optional)*
> *¼ teaspoon paprika*
> *freshly ground pepper to taste*
> *2 tablespoons shredded skim-milk mozzarella cheese*

Preheat the oven to 375°F. Lightly coat a 2-cup square casserole with cooking spray.

In a heavy skillet that has been lightly coated with cooking spray, sauté the onion and mushrooms until the onion wilts and the liquid is absorbed, about 5 minutes. Stir in the tomato and spinach. Cook, stirring, until the spinach wilts, about 2 minutes.

Transfer the spinach-onion mixture to the prepared casserole. In a small bowl, whisk together the egg, egg white, milk, mustard, parsley, tarragon, salt (if using), paprika, and pepper. Pour over the vegetables and stir gently to evenly distribute the egg mixture. Sprinkle with the cheese.

Bake, uncovered, for 20 to 25 minutes, until the top is nicely browned and a knife inserted in the center comes out clean. Remove from the oven and cool on a rack for 5 minutes before cutting into squares.

Makes 2 servings.

PER SERVING: 124 calories (34% calories from fat), 5 g total fat (2 g saturated fat), 11 g protein, 10 g carbohydrates, 2 g dietary fiber, 113 mg cholesterol, 190 mg sodium

JOSLIN EXCHANGES: 1 medium-fat protein, 2 vegetable

Chile Relleno Casserole

This is south-of-the-border comfort food and a welcome change for a weekend break-fast (and terrific for a meatless light supper). The recipe calls for low-fat goat cheese, which is available in some markets, or you can make the Lower-Fat Goat Cheese (recipe follows) ahead of time.

butter-flavored cooking spray
1 4-ounce can whole green chiles, drained
½ cup frozen chopped onion
2 tablespoons golden raisins
1 clove garlic, minced
⅓ cup shredded reduced-fat Monterey Jack cheese
2 tablespoons crumbled Lower-Fat Goat Cheese (recipe follows)
2 tablespoons minced fresh cilantro or flat-leaf parsley
⅓ cup egg substitute
⅓ cup evaporated skim milk
⅛ teaspoon hot pepper sauce, or to taste

Preheat the oven to 350°F. Lightly coat a shallow 1-quart casserole with cooking spray.

Cut the chiles lengthwise into quarters. Arrange half of them in the prepared casserole. In a small bowl, combine the onion, raisins, garlic, Monterey Jack cheese, and goat cheese. Sprinkle half of the cheese mixture over the chiles in the casserole. Sprinkle on the cilantro. Top with the remaining chiles and onion-cheese mixture.

In a small bowl, whisk together the egg substitute, skim milk, and hot pepper sauce. Pour the mixture into the casserole. Using a knife, move the chiles slightly to allow the egg mixture to flow to the bottom of the casserole.

Bake, uncovered, for 25 to 30 minutes, until the cheese is melted and bubbly, and the egg mixture is set when the casserole is shaken gently. Serve at once.

Makes 2 servings.

PER SERVING: 196 calories (18% calories from fat), 4 g total fat (2.8 g saturated fat), 17 g protein, 24 g carbohydrates, 1 g dietary fiber, 16 mg cholesterol, 339 mg sodium

JOSLIN EXCHANGES: 2 very low fat protein, 1 carbohydrate (½ skim milk, ½ fruit), 1 vegetable

Lower-Fat Goat Cheese

When we wrote our earlier collaboration, *The Joslin Diabetes Gourmet Cookbook: Healthy Everyday Recipes for Family and Friends,* we were able to purchase low-fat goat cheese in our local supermarkets and cheese shops. Finding it on a regular basis can be a problem. Recently we were thrilled to read that Anne Kupper, who has for years worked closely with Chuck Williams of Williams-Sonoma fame, has found a great way to make a very tasty low-fat goat cheese. ❡ It is made the same way as our Yogurt Cheese (page 57), and it's well worth having it on hand to spread on toasted slices of a French baguette, sprinkled with herbs, to enjoy for lunch or as a snack or appetizer.

¼ cup aged goat cheese
2 cups nonfat plain yogurt (made without gelatin)

In a medium bowl, combine the goat cheese and yogurt. Spoon into a yogurt drainer or cheesecloth-lined strainer nested in a bowl. Cover completely with plastic wrap. Chill overnight or for up to 2 days for thicker cheese. Discard the whey. Transfer the drained cheese to a covered container and chill. Use within 7 days.

Makes about 1¼ cups cheese.

PER 2-TABLESPOON SERVING: 28 calories (29% calories from fat), 1 g total fat (1 g saturated fat), 4 g protein, 2 g carbohydrates, 0 g dietary fiber, 4 mg cholesterol, 48 mg sodium

JOSLIN EXCHANGES: ½ very low fat protein

Creole Egg Casserole

Serve this New Orleans–style dish over toast points made from two slices of good-quality whole wheat bread. Add coffee and fresh fruit, and you have a breakfast fit for a Mardi Gras reveler.

butter-flavored cooking spray
1 tablespoon frozen chopped onion
2 button mushrooms, sliced
½ cup chopped no-salt-added canned tomatoes, drained
1 teaspoon capers
1 cup egg substitute
⅛ teaspoon garlic powder
⅛ teaspoon hot pepper sauce, or to taste

Coat a microwave-safe casserole with cooking spray. Add the onion and mush-rooms. Cook, covered, on HIGH for 1 minute. Add the tomatoes and capers. Cook, covered, on HIGH for 3 minutes, stirring once. Stir in the egg substitute, garlic pow-der, and hot pepper sauce. Cook, uncovered, at MEDIUM power for 3 minutes, un-til the eggs are almost set and puffed.

Let stand at room temperature for a minute or two, until the mixture is com-pletely set. Serve immediately.

Makes 2 servings.

PER SERVING: 76 calories (2% calories from fat), <1 g total fat (trace saturated fat), 13 g protein, 6 g carbohydrates, 1 g dietary fiber, 0 cholesterol, 262 mg sodium

JOSLIN EXCHANGES: 2 very low fat protein, 1 vegetable

Eggs Florentine

This simple brunch or lunch dish becomes company worthy when grilled tomato slices, grilled mushrooms, and smoked salmon are added to the menu.

butter-flavored cooking spray
2 scallions (white part plus 2 inches of green), chopped
⅔ cup frozen chopped spinach, thawed and well drained
1 cup egg substitute
2 tablespoons fat-free sour cream
1 teaspoon chopped fresh thyme or ¼ teaspoon crushed dried
freshly ground pepper to taste

Lightly coat a nonstick 8- or 9-inch sauté pan with cooking spray. Sauté the scal-lions over medium-high heat for 1 minute. Add the spinach and cook, stirring, for another minute, until the mixture is well combined.

Add the egg substitute, sour cream, thyme, and pepper to the pan. Cook over medium heat, stirring gently, until the sour cream melts and the eggs are set and soft, 2½ to 3 minutes. Do not overcook. Serve immediately.

Makes 2 servings.

PER SERVING: 99 calories (2% calories from fat), <1 g total fat (trace saturated fat), 15 g protein, 9 g carbohydrates, 2 g dietary fiber, 0 cholesterol, 266 mg sodium

JOSLIN EXCHANGES: 2 very low fat protein, 1 vegetable

Scrambled Eggs with Cream Cheese and Herbs

Just before serving these scrambled eggs enriched with cream cheese, we add sour cream and herbs. The trick to the best scrambled eggs is slow cooking so they don't dry out. ❡ We used snipped fresh chives and tarragon as the herbs, but fresh basil, chervil, or flat-leaf parsley, or a combination of all three would also be excellent.

1 cup egg substitute
2 ounces fat-free cream cheese, cut into small pieces
freshly ground pepper to taste
butter-flavored cooking spray
2 tablespoons fat-free sour cream
1 teaspoon snipped chives
1 teaspoon chopped fresh tarragon or ¼ teaspoon crushed dried

Combine the egg substitute, cream cheese, and pepper in a medium bowl. Lightly coat a heavy nonstick skillet with the cooking spray. Add the egg mixture and cook over medium-low heat until the eggs are softly set. Gently lift the cooked portion with a wide spatula to allow the uncooked eggs to flow underneath. Stir in the sour cream and herbs. Serve immediately.

Makes 2 servings.

PER SERVING: 102 calories (0% calories from fat), trace total fat (trace saturated fat), 17 g protein, 6 g carbohydrates, 0 dietary fiber, 2 mg cholesterol, 348 mg sodium

JOSLIN EXCHANGES: 2 very low fat protein, ½ carbohydrate (½ bread/starch)

Yogurt Sundaes with Fresh Fruit Salsa

Sure to refresh your mind and renew your body for the day ahead, these yogurt sundaes are as stimulating visually as they are to the palate. The sundaes can be made with almost any fruit in season. Check the Joslin Exchanges (page 255) to determine the amounts to use so that your portion totals 1½ fruit exchanges. Here is our favorite combination.

> ¼ cup ripe blackberries, cut in half
> ¼ cup sliced fresh strawberries
> 6 green seedless grapes, halved
> 2 small ripe apricots, pitted and cut into 8 wedges
> 1 large ripe red plum, pitted and cut into 8 wedges
> 1 tablespoon fresh lemon juice
> 1 teaspoon sugar substitute (optional)
> 1 tablespoon minced fresh mint or cilantro
> 1½ cups plain nonfat yogurt

In a small bowl, combine the fruit, lemon juice, sugar substitute (if used), and mint. Toss lightly to mix.

Starting with a spoonful of the fruit mixture, make alternating layers of fruit and yogurt in a large goblet or tall glass, ending with fruit. Eat at once or cover with plastic wrap and refrigerate overnight.

Makes 2 servings.

PER SERVING: 186 calories (3% calories from fat), 1 g total fat (0.1 g saturated fat), 12 g protein, 35 g carbohydrates, 3 g dietary fiber, 0 cholesterol, 151 mg sodium

JOSLIN EXCHANGES: 2½ carbohydrate (1½ fruit, 1 skim milk)

Breakfast Banana Split

Wake up to a healthy version of everyone's favorite soda fountain specialty. Here we've substituted protein-rich nonfat cottage cheese for the ice cream and a naturally sweet syrup of pureed raspberries for the chocolate sauce. ❡ To keep breakfast preparation to a minimum, section the orange and puree the raspberries the night before, and store in the refrigerator until ready to use.

> 1 medium ripe banana, peeled and cut in half lengthwise
> ½ cup nonfat cottage cheese
> 1 medium navel orange, peeled and sectioned
> ½ cup fresh raspberries

Place 1 banana half in each of 2 shallow soup bowls or banana split dishes. Top each banana with ¼ cup of cottage cheese. Arrange the orange sections over and around the cottage cheese.

Puree the raspberries in a food processor or blender until smooth. Drizzle over the fruit and cottage cheese. Serve at once.

Makes 2 servings.

PER SERVING: 140 calories (3% calories from fat), <1 g total fat (0.1 g saturated fat), 9 g protein, 27 g carbohydrates, 4 g dietary fiber, 5 mg cholesterol, 186 mg sodium

JOSLIN EXCHANGES: 1 very low fat protein, 2 carbohydrate (2 fruit)

Cheese Blini with Strawberries

Blini—small yeast-raised buckwheat pancakes—hail from Russia and are traditionally served with caviar and sour cream or smoked salmon. Here we modify their use to serve for brunch or lunch, but another time you can make small blini and serve them with smoked salmon and fat-free sour cream for appetizers, checking the Joslin Diabetes Exchange List for Meal Planning (page 249) for the additional exchanges.

Blini:

½ cup nonfat pancake mix
¼ cup egg substitute
2 to 6 tablespoons water

Cheese mixture:

½ cup fat-free cottage cheese
¼ cup egg substitute
¼ teaspoon vanilla extract
½ teaspoon grated orange zest
½ teaspoon sugar
½ to 1 packet sugar substitute to taste
butter-flavored cooking spray

4 teaspoons fat-free sour cream
4 strawberries with stems

Preheat the broiler.

In a 1-cup liquid measuring cup, combine the pancake mix, egg substitute, and enough water to form a batter with the consistency of whole milk. Set aside.

Press the cheese through a fine sieve to remove any lumps. Add the egg substitute, vanilla extract, orange zest, sugar, and sugar substitute.

Coat a small nonstick sauté pan with cooking spray and heat over high heat until hot. Pour ¼ of the blini mixture into the pan, swirling it around to cover the pan and returning any excess back to the measuring cup. Lower the heat to medium-high and cook until the bottom is browned, about 30 seconds. Turn and brown the other side for another few seconds. Place cooked blini on a cookie sheet and keep warm. Repeat the process, making 3 more blini.

Spread ¼ of the cheese mixture on each blini and place under the broiler for 2 minutes, or until heated through. Fold each blini in half. Top with sour cream and a strawberry.

Makes 2 servings.

PER SERVING: 208 calories (5% calories from fat), 1 g total fat (0.2 g saturated fat), 17 g protein, 34 g carbohydrates, 4 g dietary fiber, 5 mg cholesterol, 510 mg sodium

JOSLIN EXCHANGES: 1½ very low fat protein, 2 carbohydrate (2 bread/starch)

Baked Apples with Yogurt and Almonds

Baking apples in the microwave makes them easy to enjoy anytime. Select firm apples that are deeply colored for the variety you are buying and that smell fresh, not musty. ❡ For baking select a variety that will remain firm when cooked. With all the new apple varieties in the market, we suggest Baldwin, Gala, Granny Smith, Gravenstein, or Jonathan for this recipe.

About Our Microwave Recipes

Our recipes were tested on HIGH or full power at 650 to 700 watts in a carousel microwave and a noncarousel microwave, using microwave-safe containers.

Since microwave ovens vary significantly by manufacturer and model, you'll need to determine the power of your oven from the manufacturer's instruction manual. If your microwave is less or more powerful (the newer models are 800 to 900 watts), *add or deduct 15 seconds per minute per 100 watts of power difference.* Watch the dish carefully and be sure to rotate it occasionally while cooking if your oven does not have a carousel.

2 medium tart apples, cored and peeled ⅓ of the way down
1 4-inch slice of orange rind, cut into thin matchsticks
1 teaspoon reduced-fat margarine
½ fresh lemon
½ teaspoon ground cinnamon, or to taste
½ teaspoon sugar substitute
2 tablespoons plain nonfat yogurt
1 teaspoon slivered almonds

Place the cored and partially peeled apples in a microwave-safe dish. Stuff the apples with orange rind sticks and top with margarine. Rub the pared flesh of the apple with the lemon, squeezing some lemon juice over each apple if you desire. Sprinkle with cinnamon and sugar substitute.

Fill the dish with water ⅓ of the way up the sides of the apples. Cover with plastic wrap and cook in the microwave for 4 to 5 minutes on HIGH.

Remove the plastic wrap carefully because steam may have built up. Place the apples on serving plates. Top each apple with the yogurt and almond slivers.

Makes 2 servings.

PER SERVING: 145 calories (14% calories from fat), 3 g total fat (0.3 g saturated fat), 2 g protein, 32 g carbohydrates, 5 g dietary fiber, 0 cholesterol, 38 mg sodium

JOSLIN EXCHANGES: 2 carbohydrate (2 fruit)

Breakfast Pizza

If you want to prepare a special treat for breakfast, try this fanciful fruit pizza. In the spring and summer, make it with seasonal fresh fruit. In winter, when fruits are limited in selection, combine fresh with frozen. This makes a beautiful buffet dish and is naturally sweet enough to serve as a light dessert.

2 6½-inch 98% fat-free flour tortillas
2 tablespoons fat-free cream cheese
2 tablespoons fat-free sour cream
1 cup coarsely chopped fresh fruit, such as strawberries, whole blueberries, peaches,
*   and pineapple*
¼ teaspoon ground cinnamon
1 teaspoon light brown sugar
butter-flavored cooking spray

Preheat the broiler. Place the tortillas on an ungreased nonstick cookie sheet.

In a small bowl, combine the cream cheese and sour cream, mixing until smooth. Spread evenly on top of the tortillas, leaving a thin border around the edge.

Place the fruit on top of the cheese in a decorative manner. Sprinkle with cinnamon and brown sugar. Lightly coat with cooking spray.

Broil for 2 minutes, until the fruit is heated and the edges of the tortillas begin to brown. Cut into wedges and serve immediately.

Makes 2 servings.

PER SERVING: 163 calories (4% calories from fat), <1 g total fat (0 saturated fat), 6 g protein, 31 g carbohydrates, 6 g dietary fiber, 1 mg cholesterol, 94 mg sodium

JOSLIN EXCHANGES: 2 carbohydrate (1 bread/starch, 1 fruit)

Breakfast Cod with Grapefruit and Horseradish Sauce

It never occurred to us to serve cod for breakfast until a recent visit to New York, when a similar cod dish was offered on the breakfast menu at one of Manhattan's best hotels. This is a particularly appetizing way to start the day.

butter-flavored cooking spray
1 large shallot, thinly sliced
½ cup fresh grapefruit juice
2 tablespoons water
⅛ teaspoon fennel seeds, bruised with the side of a spoon
2 4-ounce cod fillets
¼ cup fresh or frozen no-sugar-added grapefruit sections
¼ cup plain nonfat yogurt
1 teaspoon prepared horseradish, or to taste

Lightly coat a nonstick sauté pan with cooking spray. Add the shallot and cook over medium-low heat until wilted, about 4 minutes.

Stir in the grapefruit juice, water, and bruised fennel seeds. Bring to a boil. Add the cod fillets, lower the heat, cover, and simmer for 8 to 10 minutes, until opaque throughout and the sections just begin to separate. Do not overcook.

With a slotted spatula, carefully transfer the fillets to serving plates. Keep warm. Bring the liquid in the sauté pan to a boil and add the grapefruit sections. Boil for 30 seconds. Using a slotted spoon, transfer to the serving plates.

In a small bowl, combine the yogurt and horseradish. Serve alongside the cod fillets to spoon over the dish.

Makes 2 servings.

PER SERVING: 152 calories (6% calories from fat), 1 g total fat (0.2 g saturated fat), 23 g protein, 12 g carbohydrates, 1 g dietary fiber, 49 mg cholesterol, 89 mg sodium

JOSLIN EXCHANGES: 3 very low fat protein, 1 carbohydrate (1 fruit)

Turkey Hash

Years ago the *Los Angeles Times* printed a recipe for chicken hash that was served at the Ritz Carlton Hotels. The recipe called for heavy cream and egg yolks, resulting in a wonderfully delicious hash that was served with poached eggs. At that time we could and did enjoy the dish, but today our slimmed-down version better fits our special diet. ❡ Although we use turkey, you can substitute chicken if you like. If the turkey or chicken is left over and already cooked, add it along with the milk and egg substitute mixture.

1 teaspoon canola oil
1 cup frozen hash brown potatoes
¼ cup frozen chopped onion
2 tablespoons minced red bell pepper
½ pound turkey cutlets, cut into small cubes
¼ cup skim milk
2 tablespoons egg substitute
¼ teaspoon crushed dried thyme
½ tablespoon Worcestershire sauce
salt (optional)
freshly ground pepper to taste

In a large nonstick skillet, heat the oil over medium-high heat. Add the potatoes, onion, and bell pepper. Sauté for 10 minutes, stirring frequently, until the potatoes begin to soften. Add the turkey pieces and cook, stirring frequently, for another 5 minutes.

In a small bowl, whisk together the skim milk, egg substitute, thyme, Worcestershire sauce, salt (if used), and pepper. Pour over the potato-turkey mixture and lower the heat. (At this point, no longer stir the mixture). Cook until the milk mixture has been absorbed, about 3 to 4 minutes, and a crust has formed on the bottom of the hash. Turn the hash over and cook until the other side is browned, about 3 minutes. Serve at once.

Makes 2 servings.

PER SERVING: 336 calories (32% calories from fat), 12 g total fat (4.0 g saturated fat), 32 g protein, 26 g carbohydrates, 2 g dietary fiber, 70 mg cholesterol, 170 mg sodium

JOSLIN EXCHANGES: 4 very low fat protein, 1½ carbohydrate (1½ bread/starch)

Texas Chicken Sausage Patties with Grits

It's really easy to make your own sausage. This rendition has a wonderful fresh flavor without the preservatives of store-bought sausage. You will need to own a food processor in order to grind the chicken breast or you can ask your store butcher to grind it for you. You can substitute an equal amount of boneless turkey fillets, with little change in nutrient value and no change in exchanges. ❡ If you're a Texan by birth or by heart, you'll serve this with some hot salsa alongside.

Chicken sausage:

1 6-ounce boneless, skinless chicken breast, cut into 1-inch cubes
1 large egg white
½ slice whole wheat bread, cut into 1-inch cubes
2 tablespoons skim milk
2 scallions (white part only), finely minced
2 tablespoons finely minced cilantro or flat-leaf parsley
¼ teaspoon chili powder
⅛ teaspoon ground cumin
salt (optional)
freshly ground pepper to taste
butter-flavored cooking spray

Grits:

1 cup water
¼ cup quick-cooking grits
1 teaspoon reduced-fat margarine

In a food processor fitted with a steel blade, finely chop the chicken using the pulse feature. Add the egg white and continue to pulse until the mixture combines.

In a medium bowl, combine the bread cubes and milk. Let stand for 2 to 3 minutes to allow the bread to absorb the milk. Add the chicken mixture and remaining sausage ingredients. Combine well. Remove from the bowl and, using your hands (it helps to dip your hands in water first to avoid sticking), form 4 round patties of equal size. (This can be done the night before, covered with plastic wrap, and refrigerated until ready to cook.)

Lightly coat a heavy-bottomed skillet with cooking spray. Add the sausage patties and sauté until golden on both sides, about 4 to 5 minutes per side.

Meanwhile, in a 4-cup microwave-safe bowl or measuring cup, combine the water and grits, stirring well. Microwave on HIGH for 3 to 4 minutes, or until the grits are thick when stirred.

To serve, arrange 2 sausage patties on each of 2 serving plates. Place a dollop of grits alongside, top with margarine, and serve immediately.

Makes 2 servings.

PER SERVING: 212 calories (13% calories from fat), 3 g total fat (0.6 g saturated fat), 24 g protein, 21 g carbohydrates, 1 g dietary fiber, 50 mg cholesterol, 162 mg sodium

JOSLIN EXCHANGES: 3 very low fat protein, 1½ carbohydrate (1½ bread/starch)

Bagel Thins with Smoked Salmon Cream Cheese

Sunday morning to us often means noshing on bagels with a smoked salmon cheese spread while we ponder the *New York Times* crossword puzzle or book review section. ⸿ This recipe for a special breakfast or brunch can also be doubled or tripled and used for hors d'oeuvres at a party. You can use almost any kind of bagel; we just happen to be partial to pumpernickel.

butter-flavored cooking spray
2 3-ounce pumpernickel bagels, each sliced crosswise into 4 thin slices
2 ounces fat-free cream cheese
2 tablespoons fat-free sour cream
2 ounces smoked Nova Scotia salmon, chopped
1 teaspoon snipped fresh chives
½ teaspoon grated lemon zest
1 teaspoon fresh lemon juice
freshly ground pepper to taste

Preheat the oven to 450°F. Lightly coat a nonstick cookie sheet with cooking spray.

Place the bagel slices on the cookie sheet in a single layer. Lightly coat each slice with cooking spray and bake for 5 to 8 minutes, until crisp and lightly browned, turning once.

While the bagels are baking, combine the remaining ingredients in a decorative small bowl.

Serve the warm bagel thins on a plate with the smoked salmon spread.

Makes 2 servings.

PER SERVING: 292 calories (5% calories from fat), 2 g total fat (0.2 g saturated fat), 20 g protein, 53 g carbohydrates, 8 g dietary fiber, 12 mg cholesterol, 891 mg sodium (see Note)

JOSLIN EXCHANGES: 1½ very low fat protein, 3½ carbohydrate (3½ bread/starch)

Note: This recipe is not recommended for sodium-restricted diets except for occasional use.

{ Cereals and Other Starches }

Spiced Apples with Low-Fat Granola and Yogurt

The fragrant aroma of these apples cooking on the stove is sure to get sleepyheads out of bed.

1 large Granny Smith apple, cored and thinly sliced
¼ cup unsweetened apple juice
1 teaspoon fresh lemon juice
¼ teaspoon grated lemon zest
½ teaspoon ground cinnamon
¼ teaspoon ground ginger
⅛ teaspoon ground allspice
2 tablespoons plain nonfat yogurt
¼ cup low-fat granola

In a small saucepan, combine the apple, apple juice, lemon juice, lemon zest, cinnamon, ginger, and allspice. Bring to a boil. Lower the heat, partially cover, and simmer until the apples are tender, about 8 to 10 minutes.

Spoon the apples with their sauce into 2 cereal bowls, dividing equally. Dollop with the yogurt and sprinkle with granola. Serve at once.

Makes 2 servings.

PER SERVING: 134 calories (8% calories from fat), 1 g total fat (0.1 g saturated fat), 2 g protein, 31 g carbohydrates, 3 g dietary fiber, 0 cholesterol, 36 mg sodium

JOSLIN EXCHANGES: 2 carbohydrate (1 bread/starch, 1 fruit)

Homemade Muesli

Whenever we travel in Europe, we're intrigued by the many versions of muesli (a protein-rich European breakfast cereal) offered at breakfast buffets. Unlike granola, muesli grains are eaten uncooked, and most versions are very sweet. Our recipe is less sweet and quite tasty. Serve it with skim milk or mixed into plain yogurt. ❡ If you like a "more cooked" flavor, you can toast the rolled oats in a single layer in a shallow baking dish in a 350°F oven for fifteen to twenty minutes, shaking the pan every so often to ensure even toasting.

½ cup rolled oats (toasting optional)
¼ cup rolled wheat (wheat flakes)
2 tablespoons oat bran
2 tablespoons wheat bran
2 tablespoons wheat germ
1 tablespoon golden raisins
1 tablespoon diced dried apricots
1 tablespoon sliced almonds

In a medium bowl, combine all the ingredients. Store in a tightly covered container until ready to use.

Makes 2 servings.

PER SERVING: 200 calories (17% calories from fat), 4 g total fat (0.6 g saturated fat), 8 g protein, 38 g carbohydrates, 7 g dietary fiber, 0 cholesterol, 3 mg sodium

JOSLIN EXCHANGES: 2½ carbohydrate (2 bread/starch, ½ fruit), 1 fat

Orange-Scented Brown Rice with Peaches and Milk

Topped with slices of luscious ripe peaches, brown rice makes a fine hot breakfast cereal. For added flavor interest, we've lightly scented the rice with orange as it cooks.

⅔ cup water
½ cup quick-cooking brown rice
½ tablespoon grated orange zest
¼ teaspoon salt (optional)
1 teaspoon reduced-fat margarine
1 medium ripe peach, peeled and sliced
ground cinnamon for sprinkling
ground nutmeg for sprinkling
½ cup skim milk

In a small saucepan, bring the water to a rapid boil over high heat. Stir in the brown rice, zest, and salt (if using). Lower the heat, cover, and simmer for 10 minutes, or until the water is absorbed. Remove from the heat and fluff the rice with a fork.

Spoon the hot rice into 2 cereal bowls and top each serving with half of the margarine and half of the peach slices. Sprinkle with cinnamon and nutmeg to taste. Serve at once with the milk in a pitcher.

Makes 2 servings.

PER SERVING: 136 calories (14% calories from fat), 2 g total fat (0.3 g saturated fat), 4 g protein, 25 g carbohydrates, 2 g dietary fiber, 1 mg cholesterol, 58 mg sodium

JOSLIN EXCHANGES: 1½ carbohydrate (1 bread/starch, ½ fruit)

Baked Cheese Grits

This down-home Southern dish surprises Northerners, because they can't believe they're eating grits. The steaming dish will warm you on a chilly morning, or you can use the same recipe to serve alongside broiled fish or poultry for supper. (The recipe doubles or triples easily.)

butter-flavored cooking spray
3 tablespoons quick-cooking grits
½ cup skim milk
½ cup water
1 teaspoon reduced-fat margarine
¼ cup shredded fat-free sharp cheddar cheese
2 large egg whites, lightly beaten

Preheat the oven to 375°F. Lightly coat a 2-cup ramekin with cooking spray.

Place the grits, milk, and water in a 1-quart nonstick saucepan. Cook over medium-high heat, stirring occasionally, until the liquid is absorbed and the grits

Toppings for Hot Cereals

Make sure you take into consideration exchange amounts when using these toppings on your hot cereals (see Joslin Exchanges, page 249):

- fresh fruit such as sliced bananas; whole or sliced berries; slices of mangoes, apples, or pears
- dried prunes, apricots, cherries, cranberries, blueberries, currants, and raisins
- ½ teaspoon sugar, brown or white, mixed with ground cinnamon and ground nutmeg to taste
- baked or stewed fruit
- sugar-free fruit spreads and preserves
- sugar-free syrups such as maple or fruit

thicken, about 4 minutes. Remove the pan from the heat. Add the margarine and cheese, reserving ½ tablespoon of the cheese for the top. Stir the grits until the margarine and cheese have melted. Quickly stir the egg whites into the grits and spoon the mixture into the prepared ramekin. Sprinkle the reserved cheese on top.

Bake until puffed and the edges begin to brown, about 15 minutes. Serve immediately.

Makes 2 servings.

PER SERVING: 126 calories (11% calories from fat), 1 g total fat (0.2 g saturated fat), 11 g protein, 16 g carbohydrates, <1 g dietary fiber, 3 mg cholesterol, 253 mg sodium

JOSLIN EXCHANGES: 1 very low fat protein, 1 carbohydrate (1 bread/starch)

Creamy Polenta with Dried Fruits

Polenta is full of energizing carbohydrates, makes a nice change from your morning oatmeal, and can be prepared in minutes. If your store doesn't sell instant polenta, use stone-ground cornmeal.

1 cup water
1 cup skim milk
½ cup instant polenta
2 tablespoons fat-free sour cream
1 tablespoon chopped assorted dried fruits
ground cinnamon for sprinkling

In a saucepan, bring the water and milk to a rapid boil. Add the polenta and stir constantly while it cooks, about 5 minutes. Spoon into 2 cereal bowls. Add 1 tablespoon of sour cream to each serving. Sprinkle evenly with the fruits and add a dash of cinnamon. Serve at once.

Makes 2 servings.

PER SERVING: 184 calories (6% calories from fat), 1 g total fat (0.3 g saturated fat), 8 g protein, 36 g carbohydrates, 2 g dietary fiber, 2 mg cholesterol, 86 mg sodium

JOSLIN EXCHANGES: 2½ carbohydrate (½ nonfat milk, 2 bread/starch)

Twice-Baked Potatoes with Smoked Ham

Baked potato for breakfast? Sure. A 4-ounce potato has fewer than 100 calories and is rich in potassium, iron, calcium, and vitamin C. ❡ Fortified with a little protein from shredded low-fat ham and nonfat yogurt, and lower-fat goat cheese, these stuffed potatoes are a soul-satisfying way to start a busy day. Look for Yukon Gold potatoes in your market for this recipe. These beauties are buttery in their appearance and flavor—without the butter!

2 4-ounce Yukon Gold potatoes, well scrubbed
2 tablespoons nonfat plain yogurt
1 ounce low-fat smoked ham, cut into thin slivers
2 tablespoons Lower-Fat Goat Cheese (page 33), crumbled
salt (optional)
freshly ground pepper to taste
paprika for garnish (optional)
chopped parsley for garnish (optional)

Pierce the potatoes with a fork. Arrange them on a double thickness of paper towels, positioning them so they divide the oven floor in thirds. Microwave on HIGH power for 11 minutes, or until soft when pinched. Turn the potatoes over once midway through the cooking time.

Preheat the broiler. As soon as the potatoes are cool enough to handle, slice off the top third of each potato. Scoop the potato flesh into a mixing bowl and reserve the skin shells. Mash the potato flesh and stir in the yogurt, ham, goat cheese, salt (if using), and pepper. Mound the mixture into the shells. Use the tines of a fork to give the tops a decorative finish. If desired, lightly sprinkle each potato with paprika and chopped parsley.

Set the stuffed potatoes in a small baking dish and place under the broiler, 4 to 6 inches from the heat, until they are hot and nicely browned on top. Serve at once.

Makes 2 servings.

PER SERVING: 164 calories (8% calories from fat), 1 g total fat (0.7 g saturated fat), 8 g protein, 31 g carbohydrates, 3 g dietary fiber, 9 mg cholesterol, 214 mg sodium

JOSLIN EXCHANGES: ½ very low fat protein, 2 carbohydrate (2 bread/starch)

Oven-Baked Potato Pancakes with Yogurt and Applesauce

Potato pancakes (latkes) are usually fried in vegetable oil or chicken fat. To reduce the fat, we bake them in the oven. These potato pancakes are nicely crisp, full of flavor, and easy to prepare. In fact, they are so good that you'll be glad there are leftovers for another meal when a starch (carbohydrate) is appropriate.

vegetable cooking spray
1 6-ounce russet potato, peeled
1 small onion, coarsely grated
1 large egg white
½ teaspoon canola oil
2 tablespoons unbleached all-purpose flour
¼ teaspoon baking soda
⅛ teaspoon ground ginger
½ tablespoon fresh lemon juice
salt (optional)
freshly ground pepper to taste
¼ cup unsweetened applesauce
¼ cup plain nonfat yogurt

Preheat the oven to 375°F. Lightly coat an 8 x 8-inch baking pan with cooking spray.

Grate the potato and place in a colander. Run cool water over it, stirring gently, until the starch is rinsed away and the water runs clear. Drain, squeezing out as much water as possible.

In a medium bowl, combine the onion, egg white, and oil. Stir in the grated potato. Sift together the flour, baking soda, and ginger. Stir into the potato mixture and add the lemon juice, salt (if using), and pepper.

Pat the potato mixture evenly into the prepared pan. Bake for 15 minutes, or until golden brown and crispy on the top and bottom. Remove from the oven and cool in the pan on a wire rack for 5 minutes. Cut into 2-inch squares. Serve 2 squares per person with 2 tablespoons each of applesauce and yogurt alongside. Cover and chill the 4 remaining squares for a second meal.

Makes 8 squares.

PER 2-SQUARE SERVING: 93 calories (7% calories from fat), 1 g total fat (trace saturated fat), 3 g protein, 19 g carbohydrates, 2 g dietary fiber, <1 mg cholesterol, 109 mg sodium

JOSLIN EXCHANGES: 1 carbohydrate (1 bread/starch)

Buttermilk Griddle Cakes with Sautéed Pears

These old-fashioned pancakes contain oat flour that you make in your food processor or blender from quick-cooking oatmeal. Topped with sautéed pears spiked with cinnamon, the griddle cakes make a perfect morning meal.

Griddle Cakes:

5 tablespoons rolled oats
½ cup unbleached all-purpose flour
1 teaspoon baking powder
½ teaspoon baking soda
⅛ teaspoon salt (optional)
1 tablespoon cold reduced-fat stick margarine, cut into 4 pieces
½ cup 1% fat buttermilk, plus up to 2 tablespoons additional
¼ cup egg substitute
1 packet sugar substitute
butter-flavored cooking spray

Sautéed Pears:

1 ripe pear, cored and peeled
butter-flavored cooking spray
1 tablespoon fresh lemon juice

ground cinnamon for sprinkling
2 tablespoons sugar-free maple syrup, warmed (optional)

Place the oatmeal in the bowl of a food processor fitted with the steel blade and process until it forms a fine powder. Add the flour, baking powder, baking soda, and salt (if using). Process 10 seconds to combine. Add the margarine pieces to the bowl and pulse until coarsely mixed.

In a small bowl, whisk together the ½ cup of buttermilk, egg substitute, and sugar substitute. Add to the flour mixture in the food processor and process until smooth. Let the batter stand for 5 to 10 minutes before cooking. (The batter should have the consistency of heavy cream; if it's too thick, thin with the additional buttermilk, adding ½ tablespoon at a time.)

When ready to cook, preheat a griddle or heavy-bottomed skillet. Lightly coat with cooking spray. Pour ¼ cup of batter for each cake onto the hot griddle. Cook until bubbles cover the top of each cake and the bottom is lightly browned, about 2 minutes. Turn the cakes with a spatula and brown the other side. Transfer the cooked cakes to a heated serving plate and keep warm.

To make the pears, cut into quarters and slice each quarter crosswise into ½-inch slices. Lightly coat a nonstick skillet with cooking spray. Add the pears and lemon juice. Cook over medium-high heat until the pears are soft but still crisp, about 2 minutes.

To serve, arrange 2 griddle cakes on each of 2 plates. Spoon the pears onto the cakes, dividing equally. Sprinkle with cinnamon and serve. If desired, offer warmed sugar-free maple syrup to drizzle over the cakes and pears.

Makes 2 servings.

PER SERVING: 281 calories (17% calories from fat), 6 g total fat (1.3 g saturated fat), 10 g protein, 49 g carbohydrates, 4 g dietary fiber, 2 mg cholesterol, 424 mg sodium

JOSLIN EXCHANGES: ½ very low fat protein, 3 carbohydrate (2 bread/starch, 1 fruit), 1 fat

Silver Dollar Apple Pancakes

These small pancakes are a hit with young and old alike. Unlike most pancakes, they don't have the characteristic bubbles that pop, announcing that the pancakes are ready to turn. You'll have to lift up the edge with a pancake turner to see if the underside is golden brown and ready for turning. Unless you're using a 12-inch pan or large griddle, you may need to make these heavenly pancakes in two batches.

> *⅔ cup nonfat pancake mix*
> *butter-flavored cooking spray*
> *1 small tart apple such as Gala, Granny Smith, or Jonathan, cored and cut into 8 thin*
> *   slices*
> *ground cinnamon to taste*
> *½ cup sugar-free maple syrup, heated*

Prepare the pancake batter with water, following the instructions on the box. Set aside.

Lightly coat a large nonstick sauté pan with cooking spray and place over medium-high heat for 1 minute. Put the apple slices in the pan and sauté for 1 minute on each side. Lightly sprinkle the apples with ground cinnamon.

Spoon the pancake batter over each apple slice just to cover. Cook over medium-high heat until golden brown on the bottom, then turn with a plastic spatula. Cook until the bottom is golden brown. Divide the pancakes between 2 plates and serve. Pass the syrup separately.

Makes 2 servings.

PER SERVING: 212 calories (1% calories from fat), <1 g total fat (trace saturated fat), 4 g protein, 53 g carbohydrates, 6 g dietary fiber, 0 cholesterol, 429 mg sodium

JOSLIN EXCHANGES: 3½ carbohydrate (2½ bread/starch, 1 fruit)

Fillings for Crepes

When filling crepes, remember that two crepes equals one serving. Make sure that you keep the rest of your meal plan and the exchange amounts in mind when selecting a filling (see Joslin Exchanges, page 249).

BREAKFAST:

- Fat-free cottage cheese mixed with fat-free sour cream and chopped fresh fruit
- Sautéed fresh berries or fruit seasoned with ground cinnamon, ground nutmeg, or ground allspice
- Smoked salmon and fat-free cream cheese with dill
- Fat-free sour cream with grated orange zest and cut sections of orange

BRUNCH:

- Chopped spinach and mushrooms
- Shellfish salad, made with fat-free mayonnaise
- Chicken salad, made with fresh fruit and yogurt dressing
- Grilled vegetables

Breakfast Crepes

The idea of crepes for breakfast conjures up visions of a slow, leisurely meal on the veranda, but these thin pancakes are so quick and easy to prepare, you can enjoy them anytime and anywhere.

> 1 cup nonfat pancake mix
> ½ cup egg substitute
> ⅓ to ½ cup water
> butter-flavored cooking spray
> 2 cups fresh berries: blueberries, strawberries, blackberries, raspberries, or a mixture,
>   stemmed and washed
> 2 tablespoons fat-free sour cream

In a medium bowl, combine the pancake mix, egg substitute, and sufficient water to make a thin batter. Set aside.

Coat a nonstick saucepan with cooking spray, add the berries, and warm over low heat, stirring gently so that they remain whole. Place the pan over hot water to keep warm.

Coat an 8-inch nonstick sauté pan with cooking spray and place over medium-high heat. When hot, add 3 tablespoons of batter and tilt the pan to spread the batter evenly over the entire bottom. Cook until the crepe appears dry and the edge is lightly browned, about 30 seconds. Turn over and cook for another 30 seconds. Turn the cooked crepe onto a towel and fold in quarters. Continue making them until you have 6 crepes.

To serve, arrange 3 crepes on each plate and cover with warm berries. Top each serving with half of the sour cream.

Makes 2 servings.

PER SERVING: 294 calories (2% calories from fat), 1 g total fat (0.1 g saturated fat), 13 g protein, 65 g carbohydrates, 10 g dietary fiber, 0 cholesterol, 552 mg sodium

JOSLIN EXCHANGES: 1 very low fat protein, 4 carbohydrate (3 bread/starch, 1 fruit)

Cinnamon-Raisin Puffed French Toast

This dish, made of traditional French toast ingredients, reminds us of a light bread pudding. Serve it with some warmed unsweetened canned fruit and a sprinkle of nutmeg. Check Fruit Choices (page 255) to determine serving size and number of exchanges.

butter-flavored cooking spray
1½ slices good-quality home-style white or whole wheat bread
1 cup egg substitute
3 tablespoons cold water
1 teaspoon ground cinnamon
1 tablespoon golden raisins
⅛ teaspoon salt (optional)
½ teaspoon sugar substitute

Preheat the oven to 450°F. Put a kettle of water on the stove to boil. Lightly coat an ovenproof 1-quart baking dish with cooking spray.

Break the bread into large pieces and arrange in the bottom of the prepared dish in a single layer.

In a medium bowl, whisk together the egg substitute and remaining ingredients, and blend well. Pour the mixture over the bread.

Place the dish in the center of a deep ovenproof pan. Pour boiling water into the pan until it reaches halfway up the sides of the filled dish. Place the pan on the center rack of the oven and bake for 10 to 12 minutes, until the mixture is just set, lightly browned, and solid in the center when pressed with a finger. Carefully remove the pan from the oven and cool the filled dish on a wire rack until ready to serve.

Makes 2 servings.

PER SERVING: 143 calories (7% calories from fat), 1 g total fat (0.2 g saturated fat), 15 g protein, 19 g carbohydrates, 2 g dietary fiber, 0 cholesterol, 339 mg sodium

JOSLIN EXCHANGES: 2 very low fat protein, 1 carbohydrate (1 bread/starch)

French Toast with Peaches

Just add a pot of good coffee and the morning newspaper to this old-fashioned breakfast. Our recipes calls for frozen no-sugar-added peaches, but during the summer you can use fresh ripe peaches for even better flavor.

French toast:

½ cup egg substitute
2 tablespoons water
4 slices French bread, cut on the diagonal ¾ inch thick
butter-flavored cooking spray

Peaches and syrup:

1 teaspoon soft reduced-fat margarine
2 cups no-sugar-added frozen peach slices or peeled and sliced fresh peaches
2 tablespoons water
¼ teaspoon ground cinnamon
¼ packet or less sugar substitute (optional)

Adventures with Fruit and Spices

Try experimenting with the spices you use with different fruits, or use lemon or lime juice instead of water with sweet fruits. Lemon juice is particularly good with berries. For example, try ground nutmeg with peaches, ground allspice with apricots, ground ginger with pears, ground cloves and ground cinnamon with plums, and ground cinnamon with apples.

In a flat dish big enough to hold the slices of bread, whisk together the egg substitute and water. Add the bread slices and carefully turn each slice, allowing the bread to soak up the raw egg mixture.

Lightly coat a heavy-bottomed nonstick skillet with cooking spray. Add the soaked bread to the skillet and cook over medium heat, turning once, until both sides are nicely browned, about 3 minutes per side.

While the toast is browning, melt the margarine in a small nonstick skillet. Add the peaches, water, and cinnamon. Bring to a boil and cook until the liquid is syrupy, about 2 minutes. Add the sweetener (if using). Remove from the heat and cover to keep warm.

To serve, arrange 2 slices of the toast on each of 2 serving plates. Top each serving with half of the peach syrup and peaches.

If desired, you can chop all but 4 slices of the peaches into smaller pieces. Surround the toast with the chopped peaches and place 2 whole slices on top of each serving along with the syrup.

Makes 2 servings.

PER SERVING: 306 calories (10% calories from fat), 3 g total fat (0.7 g saturated fat), 13 g protein, 56 g carbohydrates, 5 g dietary fiber, 0 cholesterol, 548 mg sodium

JOSLIN EXCHANGES: 1 low fat protein, 3½ carbohydrate (2½ bread/starch, 1 fruit)

Variation

French toast can be made with many frozen or fresh fruits. Remember that berries have more liquid, so the amount of water you add may need to be decreased. Heat the berries first, then add the liquid.

{ Quick Breads }

Dried Apricot Scones

Scones hot from the oven are a favorite breakfast treat around our houses, and since they go together so quickly, you don't have to wait until the weekend to make them. This recipe calls for the occasional whole egg, because egg substitute or the use of two egg whites in place of the whole egg won't make a tender scone.

1 cup plus 2 tablespoons unbleached all-purpose flour
1 tablespoon sugar
1 teaspoon baking powder
¼ teaspoon baking soda
¼ teaspoon salt
2 tablespoons cold reduced-fat margarine, cut into 4 pieces
6 dried apricots, finely diced
1 large egg
⅓ cup 1% buttermilk
Yogurt Cheese (recipe follows)

Preheat the oven to 400°F.

In a medium bowl, sift together 1 cup of the flour, sugar, baking powder, baking soda, and salt. Using a pastry blender or 2 knives, cut in the margarine until the mixture resembles coarse crumbs. Stir in the dried apricots.

In a small bowl, whisk together the egg and buttermilk until frothy. Make a well in the center of the flour mixture and pour in the egg mixture, stirring just until the dry ingredients are moistened. Do not overmix.

Turn the dough out onto a lightly floured work surface. Pat to a 1-inch thickness, adding up to 2 tablespoons of additional flour, ½ tablespoon at a time, as needed to prevent the dough from sticking. The dough should be very soft. Cut into six 2-inch rounds, reusing scraps until all the dough is used. Place 2 inches apart on an ungreased nonstick baking sheet. Bake for 12 to 15 minutes, until golden. Serve warm with Yogurt Cheese. Store any remaining scones in an airtight container.

Makes 6 scones.

PER 1-SCONE SERVING: 148 calories (21% calories from fat), 4 g total fat (0.9 g saturated fat), 4 g protein, 25 g carbohydrates, 1 g dietary fiber, 36 mg cholesterol, 292 mg sodium

JOSLIN EXCHANGES: 2 carbohydrate (2 bread/starch)

Yogurt Cheese

Not really a true cheese because it doesn't contain any rennet or other coagulant, yogurt cheese is merely thickened yogurt with the whey drained away. It is a staple in our refrigerator since it makes a wonderful substitute for fresh cheeses. It's used throughout the Mediterranean for a spread for breakfast breads.

For a different taste, you can add chopped fresh herbs (basil, tarragon, mint, garlic, sorrel, chervil, and so forth), which makes a low-fat substitute for a French Boursin cheese. Special yogurt cheese drainers are available at specialty cookware shops, but we find a coffee filter or a double thickness of cheesecloth inside a fine sieve work just as well.

Experiment with different brands of yogurt until you find one that pleases you. Just make sure it has no added gelatin or other thickeners.

2 cups plain low-fat or nonfat yogurt

Line a sieve with a coffee filter or cheesecloth. Suspend the sieve over a deep bowl. Place the yogurt in the filter and refrigerate for several hours or overnight to allow the whey to drain out. When the yogurt has the consistency of a soft cream cheese, scrape the yogurt away from the filter and transfer it to a resealable plastic container. (Discard the liquid in the bowl.) Refrigerate for up to 1 week, discarding any accumulated liquid before using.

Makes about 1 cup

PER 1-TABLESPOON SERVING WHEN MADE WITH LOW-FAT YOGURT: 12 calories (19% calories from fat), <1 g total fat (0.1 g saturated fat), 1 g protein, 1 g carbohydrates, 0 dietary fiber, 1 mg cholesterol, 10 mg sodium

JOSLIN EXCHANGES: free

PER 1-TABLESPOON SERVING WHEN MADE WITH NONFAT YOGURT: 11 calories (2% calories from fat), 0 total fat (0 saturated fat), 2 g protein, 1 g carbohydrates, 0 dietary fiber, 0 cholesterol, 10 mg sodium

JOSLIN EXCHANGES: free

Blueberry Scones

This is really a basic scone recipe that can also be made with raspberries, blackberries, or chopped peaches or nectarines. You can change the flavor by adding raisins or currants, dried cherries, or dried cranberries. (Check the Fruit Choices, page 255, for these added ingredients.) ❡ You must use a whole egg for this recipe. Egg substitute or two egg whites won't produce the same result.

butter-flavored cooking spray
1 cup plus 2 tablespoons unbleached all-purpose flour
1½ tablespoons firmly packed light brown sugar
½ tablespoon baking powder
¼ teaspoon salt
⅛ teaspoon ground nutmeg
1½ tablespoons cold reduced-fat margarine, cut into 3 pieces
½ cup fresh blueberries, rinsed
½ cup evaporated skim milk
1 large egg
¾ teaspoon vanilla extract

Preheat the oven to 400° F. Lightly coat a heavy baking sheet with cooking spray.

In a medium bowl, sift together the flour, brown sugar, baking powder, salt, and nutmeg. Using a pastry blender or 2 knives, cut in the margarine until the mixture resembles coarse crumbs. Toss with the blueberries.

In a small bowl, whisk together the evaporated milk, egg, and vanilla extract. Make a well in the center of the flour mixture. Pour in the egg mixture, stirring just until the dry ingredients are moistened. Do not overmix.

Drop by heaping spoonfuls on the prepared baking sheet, making 6 mounds. Bake for 12 to 15 minutes, until golden. Cool on a rack for a few minutes before serving hot or warm.

Makes 6 scones.

PER 1-SCONE SERVING: 147 calories (18% calories from fat), 3 g total fat (0.7 g saturated fat), 5 g protein, 25 g carbohydrates, 1 g dietary fiber, 36 mg cholesterol, 280 mg sodium

JOSLIN EXCHANGES: 2 carbohydrate (2 bread/starch)

Nonfat Corn Muffins

These muffins are like chameleons: They easily adapt to suit the occasion. Add chile peppers for a Southwestern taste or fresh or dried fruit for breakfast or as an accompaniment for poultry dishes. The recipe can be tripled and baked as corn bread in an 8-inch square pan.

butter-flavored cooking spray
½ cup yellow cornmeal
2½ tablespoons flour
¾ teaspoon baking powder
⅓ teaspoon baking soda
⅛ teaspoon salt
¼ teaspoon sugar substitute (optional)
2 tablespoons egg substitute or 1 large egg white, slightly beaten
5½ ounces 1% buttermilk

Preheat the oven to 425°F. Lightly coat 4 regular nonstick muffin cups with cooking spray. Fill any vacant spaces in the muffin tin with water to prevent scorching.

In a medium bowl, combine the cornmeal, flour, baking powder, baking soda, salt, and sugar substitute (if using).

In a small bowl, whisk together the egg substitute and buttermilk.

Make a well in the center of the cornmeal mixture and pour in the egg mixture. Stir just until the dry ingredients are moistened. Do not overmix. The batter will be thin but will thicken during baking.

Spoon the batter into the prepared muffin cups, filling almost to the top. Bake for 12 to 15 minutes, until browned and a tester inserted in the center comes out clean. Cool in the pan on a rack for 5 minutes before removing from pan. Serve warm.

Makes 2 servings.

PER SERVING: 208 calories (8% from fat), 2 g total fat (0.6 g saturated fat), 8 g protein, 38 g carbohydrates, 3 g dietary fiber, 3 mg cholesterol, 631 mg sodium

JOSLIN EXCHANGES: 2½ carbohydrate (2½ bread/starch)

Variations

The following ingredients can be added to the basic nonfat corn muffin recipe and will result in these changes:

- 2 tablespoons minced canned green chiles

  PER SERVING: 208 calories (8% from fat), 2 g total fat (0.6 g saturated fat), 8 g protein, 38 g carbohydrates, 3 g dietary fiber, 3 mg cholesterol, 631 mg sodium

  JOSLIN EXCHANGES: 2½ carbohydrate (2½ bread/starch)

- ¼ cup thawed frozen corn kernels

  PER SERVING: 224 calories (8% from fat), 2 g total fat (0.6 g saturated fat), 9 g protein, 43 g carbohydrates, 3 g dietary fiber, 3 mg cholesterol, 632 mg sodium

  JOSLIN EXCHANGES: 3 carbohydrate (3 bread/starch)

- 2 tablespoons chopped dried fruit such as apricots, currants, cherries

  PER SERVING: 233 calories (7% from fat), 2 g total fat (0.6 g saturated fat), 9 g protein, 45 g carbohydrates, 3 g dietary fiber, 3 mg cholesterol, 632 mg sodium

  JOSLIN EXCHANGES: 3 carbohydrate (2½ bread/starch, ½ fruit)

- 2 tablespoons finely chopped ripe pears or apples

  PER SERVING: 214 calories (8% from fat), 2 g total fat (0.6 g saturated fat), 8 g protein, 40 g carbohydrates, 3 g dietary fiber, 3 mg cholesterol, 631 mg sodium

  JOSLIN EXCHANGES: 3 carbohydrate (3 bread/starch)

Low-Fat Pumpkin Muffins with Crunchy Topping

These muffins are sublime, in large part due to their nicely spiced crunchy topping. Serve these on a cold morning, and you're sure to get raves. Use the leftover pumpkin to make pumpkin soup or pumpkin custard for dinner.

¾ cup unbleached all-purpose flour
½ cup rolled oats
¼ cup firmly packed brown sugar
1 teaspoon baking powder
½ teaspoon baking soda
½ teaspoon ground cinnamon
½ teaspoon ground nutmeg
¼ teaspoon ground allspice
⅛ teaspoon salt (optional)
½ cup canned pumpkin
1 large egg, slightly beaten
½ cup skim milk
2 tablespoons reduced-fat stick margarine, melted

Crunchy topping:

2 tablespoons rolled oats
½ tablespoon firmly packed brown sugar
1½ teaspoons grated orange zest
⅛ teaspoon ground cinnamon

Preheat the oven to 400°F. Line 6 regular muffin tins with paper baking cups or lightly coat the bottoms only with vegetable cooking spray.

In a medium bowl, combine the flour, oats, brown sugar, baking powder, baking soda, cinnamon, nutmeg, allspice, and salt (if using).

In a small bowl, whisk together the pumpkin, egg, milk, and margarine. Make a well in the center of the dry ingredients and add the pumpkin mixture. Mix just until the dry ingredients are moistened. Do not overmix.

Spoon the batter into the prepared muffin cups, filling almost full.

Combine the topping ingredients and sprinkle evenly over the top of each muffin. Bake for 22 to 25 minutes, or until a tester inserted in the center comes out with only a few moist crumbs attached. Cool the muffins in the pan on a wire rack for 5 minutes before removing. Serve warm.

Makes 6 muffins.

PER 1-MUFFIN SERVING: 164 calories (22% from fat), 4 g total fat (1 g saturated fat), 5 g protein, 28 g carbohydrates, 2 g dietary fiber, 36 mg cholesterol, 150 mg sodium

JOSLIN EXCHANGES: 2 carbohydrate (2 bread/starch), 1 fat

Low-Fat Granola Muffins

These are great bake-ahead muffins because they freeze quite well. On days when you don't have much time for breakfast, you can quickly thaw and reheat a muffin in the microwave, following your microwave manufacturer's instructions. Or wrap them in aluminum foil and reheat in a 350°F oven for 10 to 15 minutes.

½ cup low-fat granola
¼ cup plus 2 tablespoons unbleached all-purpose flour
2 tablespoons sugar
1 teaspoon baking powder
⅛ teaspoon salt (optional)
½ cup skim milk
1 large egg, slightly beaten
1½ tablespoons canola oil

Preheat the oven to 400°F. Line 6 regular muffin tins with paper baking cups or lightly coat the bottoms only with vegetable cooking spray.

In a medium bowl, combine the granola, flour, sugar, baking powder, and salt (if using). In a small bowl, whisk together the milk, egg, and oil. Make a well in the center of the dry ingredients and add the milk-egg mixture. Mix just until the dry ingredients are moistened. Do not overmix.

Spoon the batter into the prepared muffin cups, filling the cups ⅔ full. Bake for 20 minutes, or until lightly browned.

Remove from the oven and let cool in the pan on a wire rack for 10 minutes before removing. Serve warm, or cool completely and freeze in a large self-sealing plastic bag until ready to use.

Makes 6 muffins.

PER 1-MUFFIN SERVING: 125 calories (34% from fat), 5 g total fat (0.5 g saturated fat), 3 g protein, 18 g carbohydrates, 1 g dietary fiber, 36 mg cholesterol, 118 mg sodium

JOSLIN EXCHANGES: 1 carbohydrate (1 bread/starch), 1 fat

Apple Bran Muffins

We're always trying for a better bran muffin, and this one is a gem. The muffins are small, dense, and very moist. Serve them with Yogurt Cheese (page 57) for a great morning treat. Using egg substitute instead of the whole egg produces a muffin with poor texture.

1 large egg
2 tablespoons firmly packed light brown sugar
1 tablespoon canola oil
¾ cup 1% buttermilk
1 cup plus 2 tablespoons unbleached all-purpose flour
1 teaspoon baking soda
1 teaspoon ground cinnamon
⅛ teaspoon salt (optional)
¾ cup bran cereal (such as All-Bran)
½ cup diced peeled apple
2 tablespoons dried currants

Preheat the oven to 400°F. Line 6 medium muffin tins with paper baking cups or lightly coat the bottoms only with vegetable cooking spray.

In a medium bowl, whisk together the egg, brown sugar, oil, and buttermilk. Sift together the flour, baking soda, cinnamon, and salt (if using). Toss with the bran cereal, diced apple, and currants. Add this mixture to the egg mixture, stirring until the dry ingredients are just moistened. Do not overmix.

Spoon the batter into the prepared muffin cups and bake for 20 minutes, or until a tester inserted in the middle comes out with only a few moist crumbs attached. Remove from the oven and cool in the pan on a wire rack for 5 minutes before removing. Serve warm. Store any remaining cooled muffins in an airtight container, or freeze for longer storage.

Makes 6 muffins.

PER 1-MUFFIN SERVING: 183 calories (18% from fat), 4 g total fat (0.7 g saturated fat), 6 g protein, 34 g carbohydrates, 5 g dietary fiber, 36 mg cholesterol, 376 mg sodium

JOSLIN EXCHANGES: 2 carbohydrate (2 bread/starch), 1 fat

Spoon Bread with Canadian Bacon

In the South, spoon bread is routinely made with bacon drippings. In this recipe we use Canadian bacon, which has little fat but lots of flavor.

butter-flavored cooking spray
2 ounces Canadian bacon, cut into ¼-inch dice
⅓ cup yellow cornmeal
⅔ cup water
1 tablespoon reduced-fat margarine
¼ cup egg substitute
⅓ cup skim milk

Preheat the oven to 425° F. Coat a 1¾-cup ramekin or baking dish with cooking spray.

Lightly coat a nonstick skillet with cooking spray. Add the bacon and sauté over high heat for 2 minutes. Set aside.

Place the cornmeal and water in a small nonstick pot. Bring to a boil. Stir and cook for 1 minute, then remove from the heat. Stir in the margarine, egg substitute, and milk in that order. Add the reserved Canadian bacon. Spoon the mixture into the prepared ramekin.

Bake for about 15 minutes, until set and browned around the edges. Serve warm.

Makes 2 servings.

PER SERVING: 176 calories (32% calories from fat), 6 g total fat (1.6 g saturated fat), 12 g protein, 18 g carbohydrates, 1 g dietary fiber, 15 mg cholesterol, 242 mg sodium

JOSLIN EXCHANGES: 1 very low fat protein, 1 carbohydrate (1 bread/starch), 1 fat

Tea and Caffeine

Research has found that large amounts—more than 500 milligrams—of caffeine (commonly found in coffee and tea) can make blood sugar levels rise. Used in moderation (equivalent to two or three 5-ounce cups of drip-brewed coffee), caffeine should not cause a problem, but if you find your blood sugar levels are higher after drinking a caffeine beverage, you might want to switch to a decaffeinated product. As always, it's best to discuss any concerns with your health care team.

A drip-brewed 5-ounce cup of coffee contains 139 milligrams of caffeine. Tea contains much less caffeine than coffee.

The green tea of Japan and China has a delicate flavor since its leaves are not fermented before drying. It is the tea most filled with nutritional tannins, believed by the ancient Chinese to give long life and used by the ancient Greeks to treat colds and asthma. Two of the most popular green teas are Gunpowder and Basket Fried.

Black tea is next best and has a more intense flavor since its leaves are fermented before drying. Souchong, orange pekoe, and pekoe refer to the grades and shape of the black-tea leaves. The varieties with which we are familiar include Darjeeling, Ceylon (English Breakfast), and Earl Grey.

In taste, oolong tea falls in between green tea and black tea since its leaves are partially fermented. The most popular variety is Formosa Oolong.

To brew black or oolong teas, use 1 teaspoon to a cup of hot, but not boiling, water. Infuse the tea in a covered heated pot for 3 to 5 minutes. Remove the tea leaves, stir, and serve. To brew green tea, use 2 teaspoons of tea per cup of hot, but not boiling, water. Infuse in a covered heated pot for 2 to 5 minutes. Remove the leaves, stir, and serve. Iced tea is best brewed strong, then diluted with cold water. Store tea in airtight containers in a dry, dark place.

Don't forget the specialty herb teas that have various floral and spice tastes added. Herb tea is not an actual tea but a combination of herbs, flowers, and spices, and it contains no caffeine.

Here is a quick guide to the caffeine content of a 5-ounce cup of brewed tea and coffee.

Tea bags (black tea)

5-minute brew   47 mg
1-minute brew   29 mg

Loose Tea

Black and Oolong   5-minute brew   41 mg
Green (Chinese)   5-minute brew   36 mg
Green (Japanese)   5-minute brew   21 mg
Herb (any variety) 5-minute brew   0 mg

Coffee (not decaffeinated)

Drip-brewed   139 mg

Source: The American Dietetic Association, *Handbook of Clinical Dietetics* (1996).

Individual Irish Soda Bread

Soda bread makes a lovely addition to an English tea, offered with all-fruit jam. It's also wonderful for a special breakfast or dinner. Another time, thinly slice and toast it for a carbohydrate (bread/starch) snack.

butter-flavored cooking spray
½ cup all-purpose flour
1½ teaspoons baking powder
¼ teaspoon baking soda
4 dried apricots, minced
⅛ teaspoon caraway seeds
¼ cup 1% buttermilk
1 tablespoon egg substitute

Preheat the oven to 350°F. Lightly coat a baking sheet with cooking spray.

In a medium bowl, mix together the flour, baking powder, and baking soda. Stir in the apricots and caraway seeds. Add the buttermilk and egg substitute. Stir until dry ingredients are just moistened. Do not overmix.

Turn out onto a lightly floured board and knead for 1 to 2 minutes to form a smooth soft dough. Divide in half and shape into 2 round loaves. With a knife, press an × lightly on the top of each round.

Place the breads on the prepared baking sheet. Bake for 15 minutes, until lightly browned. Cool on a rack for 10 minutes before slicing. Serve warm or cool.

Makes 2 servings.

PER SERVING: 168 calories (5% calories from fat), 1 g total fat (0.2 g saturated fat), 6 g protein, 35 g carbohydrates, 1 g dietary fiber, trace cholesterol, 571 mg sodium

JOSLIN EXCHANGES: 2 carbohydrate (1½ bread/starch, ½ fruit)

POWER LUNCHES

When you have diabetes, lunchtime can be a challenge. A quick bite at the local fast-food restaurant or from the office vending machine may offer extra calories or fat that won't help achieve your goal of better control. Planning may be what you need! Proper noontime nourishment will help control your diabetes and effectively fuel you for the rest of your day. ❡ With this in mind, we're sharing our favorite lunches for taking to work, eating at home, or for a picnic in the park. For those who must occasionally "do lunch" at a restaurant, we have some suggestions to help you take control and assure yourself of a delicious, healthy meal.

Five Terrific Sandwiches

Lentils and Cheese in Pita

Remove the tough stems from 5 spinach leaves. Line half of a 6-inch whole wheat pita bread with the leaves. Stuff the pita with ½ cup of cooked lentils, 3 thinly sliced red onion rings, and 2 tablespoons of farmer's cheese. Drizzle with 1 teaspoon of fat-free dressing. Wrap the filled pita tightly with plastic wrap.

Makes 1 serving.

PER SERVING: 252 calories (18% calories from fat), 5 g total fat (3.1 g saturated fat), 15 g protein, 38 g carbohydrates, 7 g dietary fiber, 13 mg cholesterol, 279 mg sodium

JOSLIN EXCHANGES: 1 medium fat protein, 2½ carbohydrate (2½ bread/starch)

Tuna and Pineapple on Peasant Bread

Place 2 crisp Boston or Bibb lettuce leaves on each of 2 thin slices (1½ ounces) of peasant or other whole grain bread. (The lettuce will keep the bread from becoming soggy.) Top 1 side with 2 ounces of leftover grilled fresh tuna or well-drained water-packed canned tuna that has been mixed with 1 tablespoon of fat-free mayonnaise and 2 tablespoons of drained packed-in-its-own juice crushed pineapple. Cover with the second slice of bread and cut in half. Firmly wrap in plastic wrap and chill until time to eat.

Makes 1 serving.

PER SERVING: 245 calories (17% calories from fat), 5 g total fat (0.9 g saturated fat), 22 g protein, 28 g carbohydrates, 4 g dietary fiber, 28 mg cholesterol, 367 mg sodium

JOSLIN EXCHANGES: 2 low-fat protein, 2 carbohydrate (1½ bread/starch, ½ fruit)

Turkey Tortilla Roll-ups

Spread one 6½-inch 98% fat-free tortilla with 1 teaspoon of Dijon mustard. Cover with 2 Boston or Bibb lettuce leaves. Arrange two 1-ounce turkey breast slices, 2 small carrot sticks, and ¼ cup of alfalfa sprouts on top. Roll and wrap with plastic wrap. Chill until ready to eat.

Makes 1 serving.

PER SERVING: 216 calories (19% calories from fat), 4 g total fat (1.7 g saturated fat), 18 g protein, 25 g carbohydrates, 5 g dietary fiber, 34 mg cholesterol, 437 mg sodium

JOSLIN EXCHANGES: 2 very low fat protein, 1½ carbohydrate (1½ bread/starch)

Veggie Sandwich

Spread 1 slice of good-quality multigrain bread with 2 tablespoons of Lower-Fat Goat Cheese (page 33). Top with 1 roasted red bell pepper (homemade or brine-packed from a jar), 3 paper-thin slices of raw zucchini, 1 thin slice of ripe tomato, and 2 tablespoons of alfalfa-radish sprouts. Top with the second slice of bread. Cut the sandwich in half and wrap tightly in plastic wrap. Chill until ready to eat.

Makes 1 serving.

PER SERVING: 151 calories (18% calories from fat), 3 g total fat (1.3 g saturated fat), 8 g protein, 25 g carbohydrates, 4 g dietary fiber, 4 mg cholesterol, 236 mg sodium

JOSLIN EXCHANGES: ½ very low fat protein, 1 carbohydrate (1 bread/starch), 1 vegetable

Turkey and Slaw on a Bagel

In a small bowl, combine ¼ cup of chopped cooked turkey breast, ¼ cup of chopped green cabbage, 2 tablespoons of shredded carrot, 1 teaspoon of plain non-fat yogurt, 1 teaspoon of reduced-calorie mayonnaise, and ¼ teaspoon of dried dill weed. Toss lightly. Spoon the mixture on 1 side of a split 3-ounce sesame bagel.

Cover with the second side. Cut the sandwich in half and wrap tightly in plastic wrap. Chill until ready to eat.

Makes 1 serving.

PER SERVING: 309 calories (9% calories from fat), 3 g total fat (0.5 g saturated fat), 20 g protein, 49 g carbohydrates, 3 g dietary fiber, 31 mg cholesterol, 512 mg sodium

JOSLIN EXCHANGES: 1½ very low fat protein, 3 carbohydrate (3 bread/starch)

Five Fabulous Salads

Cobb Salad

In a covered container, top 2 cups of mixed crisp salad greens with 2 cherry tomatoes, halved; 1 radish, sliced; 3 thin slices of cucumber; 1 ounce of turkey breast, cut into ¼-inch strips; and 1 ounce of skim milk Swiss cheese, sliced into ¼-inch strips. Cover tightly. Pack a separate small container with 1 tablespoon of fat-free dressing made with mustard. When ready to serve, drizzle the dressing over the salad.

Makes 1 serving.

PER SERVING: 130 calories (17% calories from fat), 2 g total fat (0.9 g saturated fat), 16 g protein, 10 g carbohydrates, 2 g dietary fiber, 17 mg cholesterol, 474 mg sodium

JOSLIN EXCHANGES: 2 very low fat protein, 2 vegetable

Warm Spinach Salad

If you take your lunch to work, pack the items separately to assemble and microwave at the office. Take along a microwave-safe large dinner plate. When ready to eat, pile 3 cups of fresh spinach leaves, washed, dried well, and tough stems removed, onto the plate, mounding slightly in the middle. Top with 4 button mushrooms, thinly sliced; 3 thin rings of red onion; and ¼ cup of shredded fat-free mozzarella cheese.

At home, mix together 1½ teaspoons of balsamic vinegar, 1 teaspoon of olive oil, 1 teaspoon of water, and freshly ground pepper to taste. Pack in a small covered container.

When ready to eat, sprinkle the dressing over the salad. Place the plate in the microwave and cook on MEDIUM for about 1 minute, until the cheese melts and the spinach is warm but not cooked. Eat at once. (If eating at home, you can also place the salad on an ovenproof plate and pop it under a preheated broiler until the cheese melts.)

Makes 1 serving.

PER SERVING: 140 calories (31% calories from fat), 5 g total fat (0.7 g saturated fat), 13 g protein, 14 g carbohydrates, 6 g dietary fiber, <1 mg cholesterol, 411 mg sodium

JOSLIN EXCHANGES: 1 very low fat protein, 2 vegetable, 1 fat

Tabbouleh in Romaine Leaves

In a small bowl, soak ¼ cup of fine-grain bulgur wheat in ½ cup of water for 30 minutes, until the bulgur is soft and all the water has been absorbed. Fluff with a fork. Add 3 tablespoons of fresh lemon juice and 1 teaspoon of olive oil. Fluff again. Stir in ½ cup of chopped ripe tomato, ¼ cup of chopped, peeled, and seeded cucumber, ¼ cup of chopped flat-leaf parsley, 2 tablespoons of minced red onion, 1 minced clove garlic (optional), 1 teaspoon of minced fresh mint, and 1 teaspoon of minced fresh dill. Toss lightly. Taste and season with salt (optional) and freshly ground pepper. Pack into a covered plastic container and chill overnight or for at least 2 hours. Wash and crisp 3 small inner leaves of romaine lettuce. Pack the lettuce in a self-sealing plastic bag. To serve, spoon the tabbouleh on the lettuce leaves and eat out of hand.

Makes 1 serving.

PER SERVING: 216 calories (22% calories from fat), 6 g total fat (0.7 g saturated fat), 7 g protein, 41 g carbohydrates, 7 g dietary fiber, <1 mg cholesterol, 28 mg sodium

JOSLIN EXCHANGES: 2 carbohydrate (2 bread/starch), 1 vegetable, 1 fat

Black Bean Salad

In a small bowl, combine ½ can of rinsed and well-drained black beans with 1 finely chopped plum tomato, 1 minced scallion (white part plus 1 inch of green), 1 minced jalapeño chile (optional), and 2 tablespoons of minced cilantro. Toss lightly. In a small glass measuring cup, whisk together 2 tablespoons of fresh lemon juice, 1 teaspoon of olive oil, ⅛ teaspoon of grated lemon zest (optional), ⅛ teaspoon of ground cumin, salt (optional), and freshly ground pepper to taste. Pour over the bean mixture and toss again. Pack the bean salad into a covered plastic container and chill until ready to serve. Cut 1 small red bell pepper into quarters lengthwise and remove the seeds and white pith. Pack the pepper strips into a self-sealing plastic bag. Chill until ready to serve.

To serve, spoon some of the black bean salad into the cavity of a pepper strip. Eat out of hand.

Makes 1 serving.

PER SERVING: 186 calories (27% calories from fat), 6 g total fat (0.7 g saturated fat), 9 g protein, 28 g carbohydrates, 9 g dietary fiber, 0 cholesterol, 210 mg sodium

JOSLIN EXCHANGES: 1½ carbohydrate (1½ bread/starch), 1 vegetable, 1 fat

Pichi Pachi (Italian Spaghetti Salad)

In the bottom of a 2-cup shallow plastic container with a cover, arrange ⅔ cup of well-drained, cold, cooked spaghetti. Top with ½ cup of chopped fresh tomato, ¼ cup of chopped red onion, and 1 ounce of skim-milk mozzarella that has been cut into ¼-inch dice. Sprinkle with 2 tablespoons of chopped fresh basil. In a small glass measuring cup, whisk together 1 tablespoon of red wine vinegar, 1 teaspoon of olive oil, and ¼ teaspoon of minced garlic. Drizzle evenly over the pasta mixture. (Do not toss or mix at this point.) Sprinkle with freshly ground pepper to taste. Cover and chill until ready to serve. Serve cold.

PER SERVING: 292 calories (31% calories from fat), 10 g total fat (3.8 g saturated fat), 14 g protein, 37 g carbohydrates, 3 g dietary fiber, 15 mg cholesterol, 160 mg sodium

JOSLIN EXCHANGES: 1 medium fat protein, 2 carbohydrate (2 bread/starch), 1 vegetable, 1 fat

Five Great Soups

Vegetable Soup with Rice

Coat a large nonstick saucepan with olive oil cooking spray. Sauté ½ cup of frozen chopped onion and 1 minced clove garlic over medium-high heat for 2 minutes, until softened. Add ¼ cup of chopped red bell pepper, 1 cup of diced zucchini, 1 cup of drained no-salt-added canned tomatoes, and one 12½-ounce can of low-sodium chicken broth. Bring to a simmer and add ½ teaspoon of crushed dried thyme, 1 teaspoon of crushed dried basil, 1 teaspoon of balsamic vinegar, and freshly ground pepper to taste. Simmer for 15 minutes.

When the soup is done, place 1 cup of it in each of 4 freezer containers. Chill 1 to take to work the next day and freeze the rest for another time.

Meanwhile, prepare 1 cup of instant rice according to package directions. Package the rice in ¼-cup portions in self-sealing freezer bags. Chill 1 package and freeze the rest.

The next morning, reheat the chilled soup (the soup is also delicious cold) and pack it in a preheated (or prechilled if eating the soup cold) 2-cup thermos. Take the chilled bag of rice along and keep at room temperature until ready to eat. Add the rice just before serving.

Makes four 1¼-cup servings.

PER SERVING: 130 calories (10% calories from fat), 1 g total fat (0.5 g saturated fat), 4 g protein, 27 g carbohydrates, 3 g dietary fiber, 2 mg cholesterol, 60 mg sodium

JOSLIN EXCHANGES: 1 carbohydrate serving (1 bread/starch), 2 vegetable

Mexican Tomato Soup

Coat a large nonstick saucepan with olive oil cooking spray. Add ½ cup of frozen chopped onion, 1 minced clove garlic, 1 jalapeño chile pepper that has been seeded and minced, and one 14½-ounce can of no-salt-added diced tomatoes with their juice. Cook over high heat until the mixture has thickened, about 4 minutes. Lower the heat to medium and add ½ teaspoon of crushed dried oregano, ½ teaspoon of crushed dried basil, and one 12½-ounce can of low-sodium beef broth. Simmer for 2 to 3 minutes. Remove from the heat and pack into three 1½-cup covered containers. Chill 1 container for the next day and freeze the rest.

The next day, reheat the chilled soup and pack in a preheated 2-cup thermos. Break 3 low-fat baked tortilla chips into small pieces and place in a self-sealing plastic bag to sprinkle on each serving just before eating.

Makes about three 1¼-cup servings.

PER SERVING: 71 calories (16% calories from fat), 1 g total fat (0.2 g saturated fat), 5 g protein, 11 g carbohydrates, 3 g dietary fiber, 0 cholesterol, 79 mg sodium

JOSLIN EXCHANGES: 2 vegetable

White Bean, Spinach, and Red Pepper Soup

Coat a large nonstick saucepan with olive oil cooking spray. Add ½ cup of frozen chopped onion and ½ cup of chopped red bell pepper. Sauté, stirring often, for 10 minutes. Add 1 cup of frozen chopped spinach, one 15-ounce can of white cannellini or other white beans, well rinsed, one 14½-ounce can of fat-free reduced-sodium chicken broth, ½ teaspoon of crushed dried thyme, and ½ teaspoon of crushed dried marjoram. Simmer for another 2 minutes. Divide between 3 covered freezer containers. Chill 1 for the next day and freeze the rest.

The next day, reheat the chilled soup and pack in a preheated 2-cup thermos. Take along a self-sealing plastic bag containing 2 teaspoons of grated Parmesan cheese to sprinkle over the soup just before eating.

Makes 3 servings.

PER SERVING: 219 calories (9% calories from fat), 2 g total fat (1.0 g saturated fat), 15 g protein, 39 g carbohydrates, 10 g dietary fiber, 4 mg cholesterol, 336 mg sodium

JOSLIN EXCHANGES: 1 very low fat protein, 2 carbohydrate (2 bread/starch), 1 vegetable

Gingered Chicken Soup

In a medium saucepan, bring 1 cup of fat-free reduced-sodium canned chicken broth, ½ tablespoon of grated fresh ginger, and 1 minced garlic clove to a boil. Stir in ¼ cup of dried thin egg noddles, ¼ cup of shredded cooked chicken, and 1 minced scallion (white part only). Lower the heat and simmer for 8 to 10 minutes, until the noodles are cooked al dente. Stir in 6 trimmed fresh snow pea pods. Continue to simmer for another 30 seconds. Remove from the heat and serve at once or pack into a preheated 2-cup thermos. Serve hot.

Makes 1 serving.

PER SERVING: 210 calories (17% calories from fat), 4 g total fat (1 g saturated fat), 18 g protein, 25 g carbohydrates, 2 g dietary fiber, 58 mg cholesterol, 598 mg sodium

JOSLIN EXCHANGES: 2 very low fat protein, 1 carbohydrate (1 bread/starch), 1 vegetable

Shrimp Gazpacho

In a small bowl, combine 1 ounce of tiny cooked shrimp with ⅓ cup of chopped fresh tomato, ¼ cup of chopped peeled and seeded cucumber, 2 tablespoons of minced green bell pepper, and 2 tablespoons of minced red onion. Pour in ½ cup of canned low-sodium vegetable juice, ½ tablespoon of fresh lemon juice, and ⅛ teaspoon of hot pepper sauce. Stir gently to mix well.

Spoon the gazpacho into a prechilled 2-cup thermos. Place 2 tablespoons of fat-free croutons and 1 teaspoon of minced fresh cilantro in a self-sealing plastic bag to take along. When ready to serve, sprinkle the croutons and cilantro into the gazpacho. Serve immediately.

Makes 1 serving.

PER SERVING: 93 calories (8% calories from fat), 1 g total fat (0.2 g saturated fat), 8 g protein, 15 g carbohydrates, 3 g dietary fiber, 55 mg cholesterol, 112 mg sodium

JOSLIN EXCHANGES: 1 very low fat protein, 2 vegetable

The Best Restaurant Choices for Lunch

When eating lunch in a restaurant, read the menu carefully and question the waitperson if you have any concerns about the method of cooking. Look for terms such as *steamed, broiled, garden fresh, poached,* and *roasted.* Avoid the terms *fried, sautéed, panfried, crispy,* and *buttered.*

You can be more certain if a menu says a dish is "low in fat" or "low in cholesterol" that it's really true because the U.S. government now requires all restaurants to follow strict guidelines when it comes to making health and nutrition claims on their menus. Ask your waitperson for particulars. Pay special attention when something is labeled "low-fat" because frequently the chef will add extra salt or carbohydrates to correct the flavor.

Here are some healthy choices:

- Seafood or shrimp cocktail. Ask for the cocktail sauce (high-sodium) on the side. Request fresh lemon and some minced fresh herbs to sprinkle on instead.

- Most restaurants offer, or will prepare when asked, a steamed or grilled vegetable plate. If the vegetables are grilled, ask the chef to use almost no oil.

- Order a green salad with the dressing served on the side. Avoid eating the oily croutons; instead, get your carbohydrate from the fresh bread (without butter) that is served with the salad, or order fresh fruit for dessert.

- Almost all restaurants can grill or poach a piece of fish without sauce. Keep in mind your exchanges to ensure eating what your meal plan calls for.

- At restaurants, opt for stir-fried or steamed dishes and ask that the chef use very little oil and very little sauce.

- Indian restaurants offer a variety of low-fat vegetarian, yogurt-based dishes or low-fat salads. Ask your waitperson to help you with your choice. Enjoy ⅓ cup of the basmati rice for one carbohydrate serving.

- Mexican food can be low-fat. Order a steamed chicken or fish tamale with no sauce, steamed or broiled fish, or plain rice and beans (not refried). Ask for an order of *pico de gallo* (chopped tomato relish) instead of the usual sour cream and guacamole condiments.

- It's very easy to overeat at any restaurant. At the Italian trattoria, you're better off sharing a pasta dish and ordering a green salad with low-fat dressing, or ask for a bottle of balsamic vinegar to sprinkle on the salad. Watch out for pizzas with two or three cheeses and fat-laden meats such as pepperoni and sausage. If you are having pizza, share a small fresh tomato and basil or fresh vegetable pizza with another person and ask the chef to use half the amount of cheese.

Remember, if a restaurant makes a healthy claim about a dish, it doesn't have to print the nutrition information on the menu, but it must have the information available. Also keep in mind that restaurant portions tend to be much larger than standard serving sizes. When your order arrives, mentally compare it to your servings at home. Plan to leave the extra on your plate or ask to take it with you for another meal. Also remember that restaurant meals are a social event. Enjoy the company. Food is only food.

The Best Cafeteria or Fast-Food Choices for Lunch

Look for simply prepared items such as a salad (without the dressing and beware of the croutons), fresh fruit, yogurt, a cup of broth-based soup with vegetables, or a grilled fish or chicken sandwich. If you are having a hamburger, choose a regular (2-ounce) burger with lettuce, tomato, and onion. Request that the mayonnaise or "special sauce" be put on the side or use ketchup or mustard. A little mustard or a couple of dill pickle slices are much lower in fat calories. If you're on a sodium-restricted diet, ask for a fresh cucumber salad to help cut back on the sodium.

It's important to feel comfortable with your special dietary needs. You don't have to announce that you have diabetes, but it will certainly help if you share with your waitperson that there are certain foods you can't eat. It's not uncommon for waitstaff to hear a customer's meal needs special attention.

The Best Beverages for Lunch

Water (tap or bottled) with a squeeze of fresh lemon or lime tops the list.
More than just a thirst quencher, water is an essential ingredient for a healthy, attractive body. Since people with diabetes tend to become dehydrated more easily than the rest of the population, water is a very important part of their diet. The body performs best when fully hydrated, affecting the skin, muscle tone, and body functions. A glass of water before a meal is an excellent way to provide a feeling of fullness, and a second glass during the meal can be a digestive aid for some individuals.

A person of average weight should drink six to eight 8-ounce glasses of water every day. Not all water is created equal. Remember, if you are drinking bottled water, you are not getting fluoride. Also note that flavored waters may have calories, and some have added sodium. Check the label.

Other beverages to enjoy at lunch are diet or sugar-free soda, iced tea, hot tea, and decaffeinated coffee.

DINNER

{ Pasta, Rice, and Pizza }

Angel-Hair Pasta with Roasted Eggplant and Onion

Chunks of roasted eggplant, onion, and garlic are tossed with fresh tomatoes and skim-milk ricotta cheese for a quick pasta meal. We've used angel-hair or capellini pasta here, but you can also use spaghetti, linguine, fettuccine, or a denser pasta such as penne, rigatoni, or ziti.

1 small unpeeled eggplant (about ¾ pound), cut into 1-inch cubes
⅛ teaspoon salt (optional)
1 medium onion, cut into 1-inch cubes
4 whole cloves garlic, cut in half lengthwise
olive oil cooking spray
freshly ground pepper to taste
2 medium plum tomatoes, chopped
4 ounces dried angel-hair pasta
2 tablespoons chopped fresh basil
⅓ cup part-skim ricotta cheese

Preheat the oven to 425°F.

Sprinkle the eggplant with salt (if using). Let stand for 5 minutes. Combine the eggplant, onion, and garlic. Lightly coat a nonstick baking pan with cooking spray.

Evenly spread the vegetables in the prepared pan. Lightly coat the vegetables with cooking spray. Roast, stirring occasionally, until just tender and golden brown, about 15 minutes. Add the tomatoes, turn off the oven, and leave the roasting pan in the closed oven while cooking the pasta.

In a medium pot of boiling water, cook the pasta according to package directions until al dente, about 12 minutes. Drain well, then gently toss with the vegetables, basil, and ricotta cheese, using 2 forks. Divide the pasta between 2 pasta plates and serve at once.

Makes 2 servings.

PER SERVING: 358 calories (12% calories from fat), 5 g total fat (2.1 g saturated fat), 15 g protein, 66 g carbohydrates, 8 g dietary fiber, 13 mg cholesterol, 66 mg sodium

JOSLIN EXCHANGES: ½ low-fat protein, 3 carbohydrate (3 bread/starch), 4 vegetable

Linguine with Easy Clam Sauce

This is one of the nicest pasta sauces we've ever made. Since fresh littleneck clams may not be available in your market, we call for canned clams and use the steamed littlenecks for added flavor as an optional garnish. This recipe is suffient for three servings, making it a good dish for when you have an extra guest. Otherwise, you'll have a serving left for the next day.

Fresh Herbs

Fresh herbs are so essential to our cooking style that we can't imagine cooking (or eating) a meal without them. We both have large herb gardens during our long growing season. At the first sign of frost (which for us doesn't come until after Christmas), we bring the pots indoors and cut bunches of herbs from the garden to hang upside down to dry in our kitchen. For those who don't grow their own, fresh herbs are now available in almost all supermarkets year-round.

Whenever possible we have included a dried herb equivalent in our recipes for those who prefer to cook with dried herbs. Just remember that dried herbs will lose their flavor after six months. Buy small amounts and mark the date on the bottle when you first purchase it.

4 ounces dried linguine

6 littleneck clams, well scrubbed (optional)

½ cup dry white wine or water (optional)

1 shallot, chopped (optional)

2 sprigs fresh parsley (optional)

½ tablespoon olive oil

2 cloves garlic, thinly sliced

⅛ teaspoon crushed red pepper flakes

1 14½-ounce can no-salt-added tomatoes, drained and sliced ¼ inch thick, juice
   reserved

¼ cup chopped flat-leaf parsley

1 teaspoon minced fresh oregano or ¼ teaspoon crushed dried

1 6½-ounce can minced clams packed in natural juice, drained

2 tablespoons freshly grated Parmesan cheese

2 tablespoons dry unseasoned bread crumbs

In a large saucepan of boiling water, cook the linguine according to package directions until al dente, about 8 to 10 minutes. Drain and keep warm.

Meanwhile, if using fresh littlenecks, place them in a pot with the wine, shallot, and parsley. Cover the pot and steam over high heat, shaking occasionally, until the clams are open, 5 to 10 minutes.

In a large deep skillet, heat the olive oil over medium-low heat. Add the garlic and sauté until the garlic is lightly browned, 4 to 5 minutes. Stir in the red pepper flakes.

Add the cooked pasta, tomatoes, chopped parsley, oregano, minced clams, and cheese. Toss to combine and cook for another 2 minutes. If the pasta seems dry, add the reserved tomato juice as needed.

To serve, divide the pasta among 3 plates. Arrange the steamed littleneck clams (if using) on each serving and sprinkle on the bread crumbs. Serve at once.

Makes 3 servings.

PER SERVING: 313 calories (17% calories from fat), 6 g total fat (1.4 g saturated fat), 24 g protein, 41 g carbohydrates, 4 g dietary fiber, 44 mg cholesterol, 201 mg sodium

JOSLIN EXCHANGES: 2½ very low fat protein, 2½ carbohydrate (2½ bread/starch), 1 vegetable

Low-Fat Lo Mein

Asian noodles are available everywhere—and for good reason. They're quick-cooking and extremely versatile, perfect for soups, salads, and stir-fries. This low-fat version of lo mein calls for fresh Chinese egg noodles (the noodles don't really contain egg so they are labeled "imitation"), which are available at Asian markets and larger super-markets. You can also use vermicelli or angel-hair pasta. Lo mein offers an interesting contrast of texture (soft and crisp) and flavors (sweet and salty).

4 ounces uncooked Chinese egg noodles
1 cup fresh or frozen snow peas, trimmed
¼ teaspoon dark sesame oil
1 teaspoon canola oil
1 small onion, thinly sliced
1 cup thinly sliced napa (Chinese) cabbage
½ cup shredded carrot
4 button mushrooms, thinly sliced
¼ cup fat-free reduced-sodium canned chicken broth
1 tablespoon oyster sauce
1 tablespoon reduced-sodium soy sauce

Bring 2 quarts of water to a boil in a large pot. Add the noodles. Cook for 5 min-utes. Add the snow peas and continue cooking for 30 seconds. Drain well. Toss the noodles and snow peas with sesame oil. Keep warm.

In a large nonstick skillet, heat the canola oil over medium-high heat. When the oil is hot, add the onion, cabbage, carrot, and mushrooms. Stir-fry for 4 minutes. Add the broth, oyster sauce, and soy sauce. Stir-fry for 1 minute. Add the noodles and snow peas. Stir-fry until the noodles are heated through, about 1 minute. Serve immediately.

Makes 2 servings.

PER SERVING: 298 calories (13% calories from fat), 4 g total fat (0.4 g saturated fat), 12 g protein, 54 g carbohydrates, 5 g dietary fiber, 1 mg cholesterol, 642 mg sodium

JOSLIN EXCHANGES: 3 carbohydrate (3 bread/starch), 2 vegetable

Pasta with Black Beans

This recipe was given to us by Jill West, R.D., C.D.E., a consultant to Joslin Diabetes Center and the dietitian who prepared the nutritional analyses for this book. Jill makes this pasta fairly often for herself and her husband. Give it a try; we think you'll be surprised at how delectable a very low fat pasta can taste.

1 teaspoon olive oil
1 medium onion, chopped
2 cloves garlic, minced
6 button mushrooms, sliced
1½ tablespoons minced fresh basil or 2 teaspoons crushed dried
1 tablespoon minced fresh oregano or 1 teaspoon crushed dried
⅛ teaspoon freshly ground pepper
1 14½-ounce can no-salt-added tomatoes, chopped
4 ounces dried fettuccine
1 8-ounce can low-sodium tomato sauce
1 cup canned black beans, well rinsed

In a medium saucepan, heat the oil over medium-high heat. Add the onion and garlic, and sauté for 2 minutes. Add the mushrooms and sauté for another 3 minutes. Add the basil, oregano, pepper, and tomatoes. Lower the heat and simmer for 5 minutes.

While the sauce is simmering, cook the fettuccine in a medium pot according to package directions to al dente, omitting any fat and salt. Drain the pasta.

Add the tomato sauce and beans to the sauce and cook until heated through, about 4 minutes. Arrange the drained pasta on 2 plates or in pasta bowls and top each with ¼ of the sauce. Transfer the remaining sauce to a covered container and refrigerate.

Makes 2 servings plus enough sauce for an additional 2 servings.

PER SERVING: 326 calories (9% calories from fat), 3 g total fat (0.2 g saturated fat), 14 g protein, 64 g carbohydrate, 9 g dietary fiber, 0 cholesterol, 459 mg sodium

JOSLIN EXCHANGES: 1 very low fat protein, 3 carbohydrate (3 bread/starch), 3 vegetable

Linguine with Sautéed Garlic, Broccoli, and Mushrooms

Broccoli and garlic sautéed together is a popular vegetable dish in Italy. Here we add mushrooms and pasta to make a vegetarian meal that you will want to modify to include your favorite fresh vegetables in season.

2 cups (4 ounces) small broccoli florets
4 ounces dried linguine
1 tablespoon olive oil
1 clove garlic, minced, or ⅛ teaspoon garlic powder
4 ounces button mushrooms, quartered
2 teaspoons grated Parmesan cheese

Place the broccoli in a microwave-safe covered bowl. Add 1 teaspoon of water and cook on HIGH for 1 minute. Drain, refresh under cold water, and set aside.

Bring a large pot of water to a boil and cook the linguine according to package directions until al dente, about 10 minutes. Drain, reserving 2 tablespoons of the pasta water.

While the pasta is cooking, heat the oil in a large nonstick skillet. Add the garlic and mushrooms. Cook and stir over medium-high heat until the mushrooms begin to wilt, about 2 minutes. Add the broccoli and stir until the broccoli is crisp-cooked, about 2 minutes.

Toss the pasta with the broccoli-mushroom mixture and pasta water over medium heat. Stir until the liquid is absorbed. Divide the pasta and vegetables between 2 serving plates and sprinkle with cheese.

Makes 2 servings.

PER SERVING: 312 calories (25% calories from fat), 9 g total fat (1.4 g saturated fat), 12 g protein, 49 g carbohydrates, 5 g dietary fiber, 2 mg cholesterol, 65 mg sodium

JOSLIN EXCHANGES: 3 carbohydrate (3 bread/starch), 1 vegetable, 1 fat

Roasted Vegetables over Fettuccine

Selecting seasonal vegetables varies this refreshing meal, as does changing the combination of the vegetables you use. The more you experiment, the more you'll think of this as one of your favorite basic recipes. Here's a particularly favorite combination.

olive oil cooking spray
4 thin asparagus spears, woody ends snapped off
1 small zucchini, sliced on the diagonal 1½ inches thick
1 small yellow summer squash, sliced on the diagonal 1½ inches thick
2 small plum tomatoes, quartered
1 small portobello mushroom, sliced in ½-inch pieces, or an equal amount of
*   cultivated button mushrooms left whole*
4 scallions (white part plus 1 inch of green)
2 cloves garlic, minced, or ¼ teaspoon garlic powder
⅓ teaspoon kosher salt (optional)
freshly ground pepper to taste
2 quarts boiling water
4 ounces dried fettuccine
1 tablespoon olive oil
1 tablespoon freshly grated Romano cheese
fresh parsley or basil for garnish (optional)

Preheat the oven to 450°F. Lightly coat a nonstick baking pan with cooking spray.

Arrange the prepared vegetables in a single layer. Lightly coat the vegetables with cooking spray. Season with garlic, salt (if using), and pepper. Roast for 10 to 12 minutes, until the vegetables are just done, turning all vegetables except the tomatoes once.

While the vegetables are roasting, cook the fettuccine in a 3-quart saucepan, uncovered, in the boiling water over high heat until just tender, 8 to 9 minutes. Drain the pasta well, reserving ¼ cup of the pasta water, then return to the pot. Toss the pasta with the olive oil and divide between 2 serving plates.

Remove the vegetables from the baking pan and set aside. Add the reserved pasta water to the pan to deglaze the juices.

Arrange the vegetables on the fettuccine, dividing equally. Spoon the pan juices on top. Sprinkle with the cheese, garnish with fresh parsley or basil (if using), and serve.

Makes 2 servings.

PER SERVING: 322 calories (25% calories from fat), 9 g total fat (1.7 g saturated fat), 11 g protein, 50 g carbohydrates, 6 g dietary fiber, 58 mg cholesterol, 50 mg sodium

JOSLIN EXCHANGES: 2½ carbohydrate (2½ bread/starch), 2 vegetable, 1 fat

Microwave Vegetable Lasagna

Using oven-ready lasagna noodles for this recipe significantly cuts down on the preparation time. Make sure, however, that the pasta pieces do not overlap or touch. This recipe is so good that it's a lucky thing it makes only enough for two servings. No temptation remains for midnight snacking. ❧ You will have 5 ounces of tomato sauce left. Refrigerate it in a covered container to use on hamburgers, chicken breasts, omelets, or with fresh vegetables over pasta. You'll need a microwave-safe 2½-cup ramekin or casserole with sides at least 1½ inches deep.

10 ounces no-salt-added tomato sauce from a 15-ounce can
1 clove garlic, minced, or ⅛ teaspoon garlic powder
½ teaspoon crushed dried basil
½ teaspoon crushed dried oregano
¼ teaspoon fennel seeds, crushed with the back of a spoon
½ cup shredded carrot
½ cup shredded zucchini
1 cup fat-free ricotta cheese
¼ cup egg substitute
½ cup fat-free mozzarella cheese
3 oven-ready lasagna noodles
1 tablespoon grated Parmesan cheese

In a small saucepan, combine the tomato sauce with the garlic, basil, oregano, and fennel. Simmer while you prepare the vegetables and cheese.

Place the carrot and zucchini in a small bowl and combine with the ricotta cheese, egg substitute, and mozzarella cheese.

Cover the bottom of the ramekin with a thin coat of the tomato sauce. Break one lasagna noodle in pieces to cover the bottom of the ramekin. Spread ⅓ of the vegetable-cheese mixture on top. Cover with ⅓ of the tomato sauce. Continue to layer the remaining noodles, vegetable-cheese mixture, and tomato sauce, ending with tomato sauce. Sprinkle with Parmesan cheese.

Cover with waxed paper and place in the microwave. Cook on HIGH for 8 minutes, turning once. Remove from the microwave and allow the lasagna to rest for 3 to 4 minutes, covered, before serving.

Makes 2 servings.

PER SERVING: 297 calories (6% calories from fat), 2 g total fat (0.7 g saturated fat), 31 g protein, 41 g carbohydrates, 3 g dietary fiber, 3 mg cholesterol, 564 mg sodium

JOSLIN EXCHANGES: 3 very low fat protein, 2 carbohydrate (2 bread/starch), 2 vegetable

Mushroom Ravioli with Chunky Tomato Sauce

Fresh wonton wrappers, which are increasingly available in the produce section of the supermarket, make fine ravioli. Here the wrappers are stuffed with a flavorful mushroom mixture, and served with a quick-to-fix tomato sauce. As a time-saver, purchase the mushrooms already cleaned and sliced. ❡ To complete this meal just add a salad of mixed greens tossed with orange slices to complement the hint of orange in the sauce.

½ cup frozen chopped onion
6 ounces fresh sliced button mushrooms, roughly chopped
1½ teaspoons fresh thyme or ½ teaspoon crushed dried
1 clove garlic, minced
freshly ground pepper to taste
⅛ teaspoon salt (optional)

Chunky tomato sauce:

¼ cup frozen chopped onion
1 28-ounce can no-salt-added chopped tomatoes with their juice
1 medium carrot, grated
½ tablespoon dried celery flakes
½ tablespoon dried vegetable flakes
2 cloves garlic, minced
1 tablespoon grated orange zest
freshly ground pepper to taste

4 6½-inch square wonton wrappers, cut in quarters

In a large nonstick skillet, sauté the onion and mushrooms over high heat, stirring constantly, until the vegetables are limp, about 2 minutes. Stir in the thyme, garlic, pepper, and salt (if using). Cook for 30 seconds. Remove from the heat and set aside.

To prepare the sauce: In a 2-quart nonstick saucepan, sauté the onion over medium-high heat for 2 minutes. Add the tomatoes, carrot, celery flakes, vegetable flakes, garlic, orange zest, and pepper. Lower the heat to simmer and cook, stirring occasionally.

To make the ravioli: Place 1½ tablespoons of the mushroom mixture in the middle of a square of wonton wrapper. Moisten the edge with water and place another square on top. Press around the filling so the 2 wrappers seal tightly. Place the filled ravioli on a lightly floured tea towel. Repeat until all the filling and wonton squares have been used.

Bring a large pot of water to a boil and add the ravioli. After they rise to the surface, cook until tender, about 1 minute for al dente. Remove with a slotted spoon and drain. To serve, divide the ravioli between two plates and ladle some tomato sauce on top.

Makes 2 servings.

PER SERVING: 195 calories (7% calories from fat), 2 g total fat (0.3 saturated fat), 8 g protein, 41 g carbohydrates, 11 g dietary fiber, 1 mg cholesterol, 163 mg sodium

JOSLIN EXCHANGES: 2 carbohydrate (2 bread/starch), 2 vegetable

Freezing Parsley

You may have noticed that we don't call for the dried equivalent of parsley. That's because parsley is one of the few herbs that can't be dried successfully. Its vibrant color pales, and its fresh peppery flavor is virtually nonexistent when dried.

Fortunately, fresh parsley is readily available, and it freezes well. We use both kinds of parsley—the Italian flat-leaf for cooking because it holds up well to heat, and the curly variety for garnishes.

Since grit and dirt hide easily in the leaves, it's essential to wash parsley well. A quick method is to immerse it in bunches in cold water, holding the stems and swishing the leaves vigorously. Repeat if necessary. Lay the parsley out on layers of paper towels to air-dry for at least 30 minutes.

To freeze whole sprigs, place on a baking sheet and freeze. Once frozen, store in plastic bags. Use straight from the freezer, chopping before defrosting. You can also freeze chopped parsley. A food processor will chop several bunches of parsley in seconds. Store the chopped parsley in plastic freezer containers. (We find an empty and well-washed plastic peanut butter jar makes an excellent recycled container.) The frozen chopped parsley can be easily measured into spoons or cups without defrosting.

Use frozen parsley freely to add a sparkling dash of color and a faint celery flavor to almost any food.

Penne Pasta with Lemon and Basil

This is one of those deceiving recipes: It sounds too easy to be superb, but it is. In fact it's not only delicious as is for a quick meal but when served cold as the basis for a pasta salad with your favorite vegetables or colorful fruits, it makes a lovely buffet dish for entertaining.

4 ounces penne pasta
2 teaspoons olive oil
1 clove garlic, minced, or ⅛ teaspoon garlic powder
1½ teaspoons grated lemon zest
juice of 1 large lemon (3 tablespoons)
¼ cup shredded fresh basil
1 tablespoon minced fresh parsley
freshly ground pepper to taste
2 teaspoons grated Parmesan cheese

Boil the pasta according to package directions until al dente, 10 to 12 minutes. Drain, reserving 3 tablespoons of the pasta water.

In a medium pot, heat the oil and garlic for 1 minute over medium-high heat. Add the lemon zest, lemon juice, half of the basil, half of the parsley, and the reserved pasta water. Remove from the heat. Add the cooked pasta and stir until the liquid is absorbed. Fold in the remaining basil and parsley. Season with pepper. Divide between 2 plates and sprinkle with cheese.

Makes 2 servings.

PER SERVING: 268 calories (20% calories from fat), 6 g total fat (1.1 g saturated fat), 8 g protein, 45 g carbohydrates, 2 g dietary fiber, 1 mg cholesterol, 41 mg sodium

JOSLIN EXCHANGES: 3 carbohydrate (3 bread/starch), 1 fat

Bow Ties with Asparagus, Cherry Tomatoes, and Mushrooms

There are more shapes of pasta than days in the month. Here we use bow ties, but you might try pasta shaped like tennis rackets for a dinner after a match, or rabbits at Easter time. Other fancy pasta include conchiglie, shells, rotelle, and corkscrews. Try whole wheat, spinach, basil, lemon, and other pasta for their distinctive tastes and colors.

4 ounces (about 2 cups) dry bow ties
2 teaspoons olive oil
1 cup sliced mushrooms
1 clove garlic, minced, or ⅛ teaspoon garlic powder
2 scallions (white part only), chopped
¼ cup dry white wine or low-sodium canned chicken broth
8 ounces asparagus, tough ends removed and cut into 1½-inch pieces
2 tablespoons shredded fresh basil or 1½ teaspoons crushed dried
8 cherry tomatoes, halved
2 tablespoons fat-free sour cream
1 tablespoon Lower-Fat Goat Cheese, crumbled (page 33)

Cook the pasta according to package directions until al dente, 8 to 10 minutes. Drain, reserving ¼ cup of the pasta water.

In a nonstick sauté pan with a cover, heat the oil and add the mushrooms, garlic, and scallions. Cook over high heat, stirring, for 1 minute. Add the wine and pasta water. Reduce the liquid by half.

Lower the heat to medium and add the asparagus. Cover and simmer for 2 minutes, until crisp-cooked. Remove the cover and add the basil and tomatoes. Cook only until heated through so that the tomatoes keep their shape.

Return the cooked pasta to the pan and fold in the sour cream. Cook until heated through. Divide between 2 plates and sprinkle with the goat cheese.

Makes 2 servings.

PER SERVING: 382 calories (19% calories from fat), 8 g total fat (0.9 g saturated fat), 14 g protein, 63 g carbohydrates, 6 g dietary fiber, 67 mg cholesterol, 35 mg sodium

JOSLIN EXCHANGES: 3½ carbohydrate (3½ bread/starch), 2 vegetable, 1 fat

Rice Stick Noodles and Spicy Vegetables

Rice stick noodles are available in the Asian food section of your supermarket. This versatile dish can be modified to use leftover meat or poultry. Just calculate the additional exchanges (see Joslin Exchanges, page 264). ❦ Here we use only fresh vegetables because they remain crisp when cooked. It takes a little while to clean and chop the vegetables, but the dish then goes together quickly.

½ of a 7-ounce package of rice stick noodles
½ cup low-sodium canned chicken or vegetable broth
1½ tablespoons reduced-sodium soy sauce
2 tablespoons dry sherry or Chinese cooking wine
½ teaspoon canola oil
⅛ teaspoon dark sesame oil
1½-inch piece fresh ginger, peeled and minced, or ½ teaspoon ground ginger
1 clove garlic, minced, or ⅛ teaspoon garlic powder
2 scallions (white part plus 2 inches of green), chopped
4 ounces fresh snow peas, strings removed
½ small red bell pepper, chopped
4 medium fresh button mushrooms, sliced
8 ounces fresh bean sprouts
1 tablespoon chopped cilantro
⅛ teaspoon crushed red pepper flakes (optional)

Boil the rice stick noodles in a large pot of unsalted water for 3 minutes. Drain well and set aside. In a glass measuring cup, combine the broth, soy sauce, and sherry, then set aside.

Heat a heavy nonstick 12-inch skillet or wok over high heat for 1 minute. Add the canola oil, sesame oil, ginger, garlic, scallions, snow peas, bell pepper, and mushrooms. Stir-fry for 2 minutes, until the vegetables are crisp-cooked. Add the reserved broth mixture, rice stick noodles, and bean sprouts. Stir-fry until the rice sticks and bean sprouts are heated through, about 1 minute. Sprinkle with cilantro and red pepper flakes (if using).

Divide between 2 plates and serve immediately.

Makes 2 servings.

PER SERVING: 292 calories (9% calories from fat), 3 g total fat (0.5 g saturated fat), 9 g protein, 59 g carbohydrates, 5 g dietary fiber, 1 mg cholesterol, 498 mg sodium

JOSLIN EXCHANGES: 3 carbohydrate (3 bread/starch), 2 vegetable

Rotini with Eggplant, Tomatoes, and Ricotta Cheese

Today's grocery stores sell dry pasta in myriad shapes and colors. Here we've used rotini, which are short spaghetti spirals, but you can also use cappelletti (little hats), farfalle (bow ties), orecchiette (little ears), or rotelle (little wheels). ❡ If you do not have fresh basil in your garden, you can purchase it at your greengrocer—the dish really benefits from its flavor. Serve the pasta with a salad of grapefruit slices and thinly sliced sweet onions over mixed greens for a wonderful light meal.

1 10-ounce globe eggplant, peeled and cut into ¾-inch cubes
4 cloves garlic, minced, or ½ teaspoon garlic powder
4 ounces dry rotini pasta
½ cup fat-free ricotta cheese
2 small fresh ripe plum tomatoes, diced
¼ cup chopped fresh basil
freshly ground pepper to taste
2 tablespoons grated Parmesan cheese
1 teaspoon olive oil

Place the eggplant in a microwave-safe covered dish with 2 tablespoons of water. Cook on HIGH for 3 minutes. Check for doneness (eggplant should be tender but still crisp). Stir and cook an additional minute if necessary. Drain well. Gently stir in the garlic and set aside.

Cook the pasta in a nonstick pot of boiling water for 10 minutes, following package directions. Drain well and return to the pot. Fold in the ricotta cheese, tomatoes, basil, pepper, Parmesan cheese, olive oil, and the reserved eggplant. Serve at once.

Makes 2 servings.

PER SERVING: 354 calories (15% calories from fat), 6 g total fat (1.6 g saturated fat), 23 g protein, 53 g carbohydrates, 6 g dietary fiber, 10 mg cholesterol, 221 mg sodium

JOSLIN EXCHANGES: 1 very low fat protein, 2½ carbohydrate (2½ bread/starch), 3 vegetable, 1 fat

Stuffed Pasta Shells with Italian Tomato Sauce

When you're cooking for two, purchase frozen vegetables in plastic bags rather than boxes so there will be no waste. Since the vegetable pieces are quick-frozen individually, they're easy to measure out, and if securely resealed, the remainder will not get freezer burn.

1½ cups frozen broccoli cuts
6 jumbo pasta shells
¾ cup fat-free ricotta cheese
¾ cup shredded fat-free mozzarella cheese
3 ounces egg substitute
2½ tablespoons grated Parmesan cheese
¼ cup chopped fresh basil or 1 tablespoon crushed dried
1 tablespoon snipped chives

Italian tomato sauce:

olive oil cooking spray
1 small onion, finely chopped
1 clove garlic, minced, or ⅛ teaspoon garlic powder
1 14½-ounce can no-salt-added chopped tomatoes
2 tablespoons low-sodium tomato paste
¼ cup water
½ teaspoon crushed dried oregano
¼ teaspoon crushed dried thyme

In a covered microwave-safe dish, cook the frozen broccoli cuts on HIGH for 2 minutes. Drain and finely chop.

Cook the pasta shells in boiling water for 8 to 10 minutes according to package directions. Do not overcook because the pasta will cook some more after being stuffed. Drain well and place on aluminum foil to prevent sticking.

While the pasta is cooking, combine the ricotta and mozzarella cheeses, egg substitute, 2 tablespoons of Parmesan cheese, basil, and chives. Fold in the broccoli.

To make the tomato sauce: Lightly coat a nonstick saucepan with cooking spray. Add the onion and garlic. Sauté over low heat until the onion is limp, about 4 minutes. Stir in the tomatoes, tomato paste, water, oregano, and thyme. Lower the heat, cover, and simmer while you stuff the shells.

Fill the shells with the cheese mixture. Use 1 cup of the sauce to cover the bottom of a microwave-safe casserole that is just big enough to hold the pasta shells in a single layer. Arrange the stuffed shells on top of the sauce and pour the remaining sauce over the shells. Sprinkle with the remaining Parmesan cheese.

Cover loosely with a piece of waxed paper and microwave, for 4 minutes on HIGH. Turn the dish and cook on HIGH for another 3 minutes. Serve immediately.

Makes 2 servings.

PER SERVING: 424 calories (8% calories from fat), 4 g total fat (1.6 g saturated fat), 44 g protein, 56 g carbohydrate, 10 g dietary fiber, 11 mg cholesterol, 789 mg sodium

JOSLIN EXCHANGES: 4 very low fat protein, 2 carbohydrate (2 bread/starch), 4 vegetable

Low-Fat Macaroni and Cheese

Not as rich as the macaroni and cheese of our youth, this is quite tasty and satisfying—and more in line with our low-fat diets. We've used penne pasta (it's still macaroni) instead of the customary elbows and added a crunchy bread crumb topping. ❡ The recipe makes four servings, so you'll have plenty left over for another meal or a couple of lunches.

butter-flavored cooking spray
4 ounces penne pasta
1½ tablespoons reduced-fat margarine
2 tablespoons finely chopped onion
1½ tablespoons unbleached all-purpose flour
1 cup evaporated skim milk
1 cup (4 ounces) reduced-fat sharp cheddar cheese
½ teaspoon Dijon mustard
½ teaspoon paprika
¼ teaspoon salt (optional)
freshly ground pepper to taste
2 tablespoons egg substitute
2 tablespoons seasoned bread crumbs (see page 91)
1 tablespoon chopped parsley

Preheat the oven to 350°F. Lightly coat a 1-quart casserole with cooking spray.

Bring a medium pot of water to a boil and cook the penne pasta according to package directions until al dente, about 12 minutes. Drain and set aside.

In a medium nonstick saucepan, melt the margarine over medium heat. Add the onion and sauté until it wilts, about 4 minutes. Whisk together the flour and ½ cup of the milk, mixing well. Add the flour mixture to the onion and cook, stirring constantly, until well mixed. Add the remaining ½ cup of milk and cook, stirring constantly, until the mixture is thick and bubbly, about 10 minutes. Remove from the heat and add the cheese, mustard, ¼ teaspoon of paprika, salt (if using), and pepper. Stir well to combine evenly. Gradually stir about ½ cup of this cheese sauce into the egg substitute, then stir this mixture into the remaining cheese sauce.

Combine the penne pasta and cheese sauce. Transfer the mixture to the prepared casserole. Combine the bread crumbs and parsley, and sprinkle evenly over the penne. Lightly coat the crumbs with cooking spray and sprinkle with the remaining ¼ teaspoon of paprika. Bake, uncovered, until the top begins to brown and the sauce is bubbling, about 25 minutes.

Makes 4 servings.

PER SERVING: 319 calories (27% calories from fat), 10 g total fat (4.3 g saturated fat), 20 g protein, 39 g carbohydrates, 2 g dietary fiber, 56 mg cholesterol, 425 mg sodium

JOSLIN EXCHANGES: 1½ medium fat protein, 2½ carbohydrate (2 bread/starch, ½ nonfat milk)

Making Your Own Bread Crumbs

You can buy seasoned bread crumbs, but since day-old bread makes great crumbs that freeze well, it's a good idea to make your own.

For homemade crumbs, slice a 1-pound loaf of day-old French bread in half lengthwise, then cut into cubes. Preheat the oven to 300°F. Put the cubes in a shallow baking pan. Bake, stirring twice, until the cubes are golden, about 15 minutes. Remove from the oven and set aside to cool completely.

Toss the cubes with 1 teaspoon of crushed dried thyme, 1 teaspoon of crushed dried oregano, and 1 teaspoon of crushed dried basil. Add ¼ teaspoon of freshly ground pepper, if desired.

Crush the bread mixture in a food processor or blender, or place the bread in a large self-sealing plastic bag and pound to fine crumbs with the flat side of a mallet. Store in an airtight container in the refrigerator or freeze. There is no need to thaw the bread crumbs before using.

Makes about 1½ cups.

PER 2-TABLESPOON SERVING: 105 calories (10% calories from fat), 1 g total fat (0.2 g saturated fat), 3 g protein, 20 g carbohydrates, 1 g dietary fiber, 0 cholesterol, 230 mg sodium

JOSLIN EXCHANGES: 1 carbohydrate (1 bread/starch)

Risotto Primavera

Primavera is Italian for "springtime," hence the spring vegetable asparagus in this recipe. But feel free to enjoy risotto with the fresh vegetables you like during the rest of the year. As a shortcut you can use defrosted frozen vegetables when getting to the market is difficult. ❡ The high-starch kernels of this Italian rice produce a creamy texture that is a requisite for the dish.

1 cup fat-free reduced-sodium canned chicken broth
⅔ cup water
¼ cup dry white wine or an additional ¼ cup water
10 thin asparagus spears, woody ends removed
3 ounces broccoli florets, separated
1 small yellow summer squash, quartered lengthwise and cut into 1-inch pieces
3 button mushrooms, quartered
2 tablespoons frozen chopped onion
butter-flavored cooking spray
½ cup Italian Arborio or Carnaroli rice
1 tablespoon grated Parmesan cheese
chopped parsley for garnish (optional)

In a heavy 2-quart saucepan, combine the broth, water, and wine. Bring to a simmer over low heat. Add all the vegetables except the onion and cook for 2 to 3 minutes, until the vegetables are crisp-cooked. Using a slotted spoon, transfer the vegetables to a bowl. Turn the heat off under the broth mixture.

Lightly coat another 2-quart nonstick saucepan with cooking spray. Add the onion and rice, and sauté for 2 minutes over low heat. Pour enough of the reserved broth mixture over the rice to just cover. Simmer, stirring, until the liquid is absorbed. Continue cooking and adding the broth mixture in ¼-cup amounts, until almost all the liquid has been added and absorbed. This should take about 10 more minutes.

Gently stir in the reserved vegetables and Parmesan cheese. Continue cooking, adding the last of the liquid, until the rice is slightly creamy and just tender, and the vegetables are heated through, about 3 minutes. Garnish with chopped parsley if desired and serve immediately.

Makes 2 servings.

PER SERVING: 254 calories (7% calories from fat), 2 g total fat (0.6 g saturated fat), 10 g protein, 49 g carbohydrates, 6 g dietary fiber, 2 mg cholesterol, 82 mg sodium

JOSLIN EXCHANGES: 2 carbohydrate (2 bread/starch), 3 vegetable

---

For Perfect Risotto

- Don't rinse the rice before cooking. It's the starch coating on the grains of rice that gives the creamy texture.

- Use a heavy pot with straight sides and a flat bottom to ensure even cooking.

- Keep both the broth and the risotto mixture at a simmer. If the rice cooks too quickly or too slowly, it won't have the right texture.

- Start testing rice grains for doneness after 15 minutes of cooking. The exact cooking time is affected by variances in the stove, the pot used, and the humidity of the kitchen. Risotto is done when it's creamy and just tender to the bite.

- Some other seasonings to try in place of saffron are crushed dried basil, dried dill weed, curry powder, ground cinnamon, crushed fennel seed, ground ginger, grated lemon zest, grated orange zest, paprika, crushed dried tarragon, and crushed dried thyme.

Mushroom Risotto

We added dried mushrooms to risotto for a lovely lightening of the classic rice dish of northern Italy. Look for bags of the dried mushrooms hanging on a rack in the produce section of your supermarket. Seal and save the rest of the dried mushrooms for another use.

¼ cup white wine or water
¼ ounce dried porcini or shiitake mushrooms
1 teaspoon olive oil
¼ cup frozen chopped onion
½ cup Italian Arborio or Carnaroli rice
1½ cups low-sodium canned beef broth
⅛ teaspoon crushed saffron threads (optional)
freshly ground pepper to taste
1 tablespoon grated Parmesan cheese

In a small saucepan, bring the wine to a boil. Add the mushrooms. Remove from the heat, cover, and set aside.

In a heavy nonstick saucepan, heat the oil over low heat. Add the onion and sauté, stirring often, until the onion is limp, about 4 minutes. Add the rice and cook for another 3 minutes.

Meanwhile, bring the beef broth to a boil in another saucepan. Lower the heat to a simmer. Add ¼ cup of hot broth to the rice, stir, and allow to simmer until the broth is absorbed. Add the saffron (if using), another ¼ cup of broth, and the wine-mushroom mixture. Continue to simmer, stirring gently. Continue adding the hot broth, ¼ cup at a time, stirring gently, until the rice is creamy but just tender. Total cooking time should be about 25 minutes. Add the pepper and cheese. Serve immediately.

Makes 2 servings.

PER SERVING: 247 calories (12% calories from fat), 3 g total fat (0.9 g saturated fat), 9 g protein, 40 g carbohydrates, 1 g dietary fiber, 2 mg cholesterol, 114 mg sodium

JOSLIN EXCHANGES: 3 carbohydrate (3 bread/starch)

Spicy Spanish Rice

Spooned over a bed of shredded lettuce, this spicy rice salad is light and lean—perfect for supper on a hot summer night when you don't feel like cooking. The recipe calls for cooked rice that you made the night before or earlier that morning. Then it's only a matter of minutes before supper is on the table. Fill a pitcher with iced tea and offer baked fat-free pita chips for scooping up the salad.

1 cup cooked white or brown rice
⅓ cup canned black beans, rinsed and drained
1 small red bell pepper, minced
1 recipe Fresh Tomato Salsa (page 97)
¼ teaspoon ground cumin
⅛ teaspoon garlic powder
⅓ cup shredded reduced-fat cheddar cheese
1 tablespoon minced fresh cilantro
2 cups shredded lettuce

In a medium bowl, combine all the ingredients except the lettuce. Toss lightly to mix well. Chill until ready to serve. To serve, divide the lettuce between 2 plates. Top with the rice salad.

Makes 2 servings.

PER SERVING: 236 calories (17% calories from fat), 4 g total fat (2.5 g saturated fat), 13 g protein, 38 g carbohydrates, 6 g dietary fiber, 13 mg cholesterol, 234 mg sodium

JOSLIN EXCHANGES: 1 low fat protein, 2 carbohydrate (2 bread/starch), 2 vegetable

Sausage and Mushroom Pizza

For this pizza you'll need to make a recipe of Texas Chicken Sausage or purchase 4 ounces of one of the many low-fat chicken or turkey sausages available at your market. There will be two servings of pizza left for another day. Luckily, pizza reheats wonderfully in the microwave. Consult your microwave instruction manual for details.

> *olive oil cooking spray*
> *1 recipe Texas Chicken Sausage (page 42)*
> *1 11½-inch thin-crust Italian bread shell*
> *⅔ cup shredded fat-free mozzarella cheese*
> *1 small white onion, thinly sliced*
> *½ cup thinly sliced fresh mushrooms*
> *½ teaspoon crushed dried oregano*
> *2 large plum tomatoes, thinly sliced*
> *1½ tablespoons chopped fresh basil or ½ teaspoon crushed dried*
> *crushed red pepper flakes (optional)*

Lightly coat a heavy nonstick skillet with cooking spray. Crumble the prepared chicken sausage into the skillet and sauté over medium-high heat until the sausage is no longer pink. Break up the sausage with the back of a wooden spoon. Using a slotted spoon, remove the sausage from the skillet and drain on paper towels.

Preheat the oven to 450°F. Place the bread shell on an ungreased nonstick cookie sheet or pizza stone. Lightly coat the shell with cooking spray.

Sprinkle half of the cheese onto the shell. Top with the sausage, onion, and mushrooms. Sprinkle with oregano and top with tomato slices. Sprinkle with basil. Lightly coat the pizza with cooking spray. Top with the remaining cheese. Bake until the tomatoes and cheese just begin to brown and the crust is crisp, about 15 to 18 minutes. Pass the shaker of dried pepper flakes to sprinkle on the pizza as desired.

Makes 4 servings.

PER SERVING: 304 calories (16% from fat), 5 g total fat (1.5 g saturated fat), 25 g protein, 38 g carbohydrates, 2 g dietary fiber, 29 mg cholesterol, 620 mg sodium

JOSLIN EXCHANGES: 2½ very low fat protein, 2 carbohydrate (2 bread/starch), 1 vegetable, 1 fat

Grilled Vegetable Pizza

In the summer the small white eggplants available in stores everywhere make a good substitute for the eggplants called for in this recipe. For a slightly different tomato taste, you can also try substituting halved cherry tomatoes or rehydrated sun-dried tomatoes (dry-packed, not packed in oil) in place of the eggplant.

2 6-inch whole wheat pita breads
1 cup shredded fat-free mozzarella cheese
olive oil cooking spray
3 small unpeeled Japanese eggplants or 1 small unpeeled globe eggplant, sliced in
    ¼-inch diagonal slices
1 small zucchini, sliced in ¼-inch diagonal slices
2 plum tomatoes, sliced in ¼-inch lengthwise slices
¼ teaspoon kosher salt (optional)
freshly ground pepper to taste
¼ teaspoon garlic powder, or to taste
1 tablespoon chopped fresh basil

Set one oven shelf for broiling and the other in the middle of the oven. Preheat the broiler.

Halve the pita bread by using a sharp-pointed knife to cut around the edge to form 4 rounds. Arrange on a baking sheet, rough side up, and sprinkle with half of the cheese. Set aside.

Lightly coat a cookie sheet with cooking spray and arrange the vegetables on it. Season with salt (if using) and pepper, and lightly coat with cooking spray. Broil 4 inches from the heat source for 2 minutes or less, just until the vegetables begin to brown. Turn the vegetables, except for the tomatoes, and broil another 1 to 2 minutes. Remove from the oven.

Reset the oven to bake at 500°F.

Divide the vegetables among the 4 pita halves. Sprinkle with garlic powder. Top with the remaining cheese. Bake for 5 to 8 minutes, until the cheese melts and the pita edges brown. Sprinkle with basil and serve.

Makes 2 servings.

PER SERVING: 273 calories (7% from fat), 2 g total fat (0.4 g saturated fat), 21 g protein, 48 g carbohydrates, 9 g dietary fiber, 1 mg cholesterol, 867 mg sodium (see *Note*)

JOSLIN EXCHANGES: 2 very low fat protein, 2 carbohydrate (2 bread/starch), 3 vegetable

Note: This recipe is not recommended for sodium-restricted diets except for occasional use.

Three-Pepper Mexican Pizza

What could be better than a combination of two popular cuisines, Mexican and Italian? Here we make pizza with south-of-the-border ingredients. The salsa is home-made to ensure fresh taste and low sodium. Once you try it, you'll see why we hardly ever use store-bought salsa. The salsa recipe makes about 1 cup.

Fresh Tomato Salsa:

1 large tomato, diced
1 scallion (white part plus 1 inch of green), chopped
1 teaspoon lime juice
1 clove garlic, minced, or ⅛ teaspoon garlic powder
1 jalapeño chile pepper, seeded and minced
2 tablespoons chopped fresh cilantro

Pizza:

1 whole wheat pita, split in half horizontally
olive oil cooking spray
½ cup shredded fat-free sharp cheddar cheese
¼ medium green bell pepper, cut into thin strips
¼ medium red bell pepper, cut into thin strips

Preheat the oven to 450°F.

To make the salsa: In a small bowl, combine the tomato, scallion, lime juice, garlic, jalapeño (start with ½ teaspoon and increase to taste), and cilantro.

Lightly coat the pita halves with the cooking spray and place on a nonstick cookie sheet. Cover each pita half with half of the cheese. Top each with half of the salsa and half of the pepper strips. Sprinkle each with the remaining cheese. Lightly coat the pizzas with the cooking spray. Bake until the cheese melts, about 8 minutes. Serve immediately.

Makes 2 servings.

PER SERVING: 142 calories (6% calories from fat), 1 g total fat (0.2 g saturated fat), 12 g protein, 22 g carbohydrates, 3 g dietary fiber, 3 mg cholesterol, 407 mg sodium

JOSLIN EXCHANGES: 1 very low fat protein, 1 carbohydrate (1 bread/starch), 1 vegetable

TOMATO SALSA ¼-CUP SERVING: 15 calories (11% calories from fat), <1 g total fat (trace saturated fat), 1 g protein, 3 g carbohydrates, 1 g dietary fiber, 0 cholesterol, 6 mg sodium

JOSLIN EXCHANGES: Free/1 vegetable for ½-cup serving

Seafood and Tomato Pizza

You don't have to give up enjoying new-style pizza on a diabetic diet. This makes an excellent and easy dinner, lunch for company, or an hors d'oeuvre when it is cut into small squares.

1 11½-inch thin-crust Italian bread shell
1 cup shredded fat-free mozzarella cheese
2 large plum tomatoes, thinly sliced
1½ tablespoons chopped fresh basil or ½ tablespoon crushed dried
4 ounces bay scallops
4 ounces medium shrimp, shelled, deveined, and cut in half lengthwise
⅛ teaspoon garlic powder
½ tablespoon grated Parmesan cheese
olive oil cooking spray

Preheat the oven to 450°F.

Place the bread shell on an ungreased nonstick cookie sheet. Sprinkle with the mozzarella cheese, leaving a 1-inch border around the rim. Place the tomato slices in concentric circles on top of the cheese. Sprinkle with basil. Arrange the scallops and shrimp over the top. Sprinkle with garlic powder and Parmesan cheese. Lightly coat the top of the pizza with cooking spray.

Bake the pizza for 10 to 12 minutes, until the seafood is cooked through and the top is browned. Remove from the oven and cut into 8 wedges.

Makes two 2-wedge servings with 4 wedges left over for reheating for lunch the next day.

PER SERVING: 300 calories (15% calories from fat), 5 g total fat (1.4 g saturated fat), 26 g protein, 35 g carbohydrates, 1 g dietary fiber, 57 mg cholesterol, 732 mg sodium

JOSLIN EXCHANGES: 3 very low fat protein, 2 carbohydrate (2 bread/starch), 1 vegetable

Note: Alternatives to the Italian bread shell include 1 medium pita bread, 2 tortillas, or 1 whole English muffin for individual servings.

Southwestern Pizza

This open-faced quesadilla takes on some Italian flavor to pair with Shrimp Gazpacho (page 72) for a light supper.

1 10-inch 98% fat-free flour tortilla
½ cup shredded part-skim mozzarella cheese
½ cup finely chopped plum tomatoes
2 tablespoons minced pickled jalapeño slices
3 scallions (white part plus 1 inch of green), thinly sliced
¼ teaspoon crushed dried oregano
2 tablespoons chopped fresh basil
1 tablespoon grated Parmesan cheese
fat-free sour cream (optional)

Preheat the broiler.

Place the tortilla on a nonstick baking sheet. Top evenly with the mozzarella cheese, then sprinkle evenly with the remaining ingredients except the sour cream.

Broil 4 to 6 inches from the heat source until the cheese melts and the edge of the tortilla is crisp and lightly browned. Cut into wedges. Pass the sour cream (if using) to spoon on individual servings.

Makes 2 servings.

PER SERVING: 178 calories (30% from fat), 6 g total fat (3.7 g saturated fat), 12 g protein, 22 g carbohydrates, 4 g dietary fiber, 18 mg cholesterol, 572 mg sodium

JOSLIN EXCHANGES: 1 medium-fat protein, 1 carbohydrate (1 bread/starch), 1 vegetable

Fresh Tomato Basil Pizza

When summer tomatoes are available and fresh basil abounds in your garden, this pizza is perfect for a light dinner, with plenty remaining for lunch the next day. Use plum tomatoes when the other tomatoes in the market are not flavorful.

1 10-ounce thin-crust pizza shell
olive oil cooking spray
2 scallions (white part plus 1 inch of green), chopped
1 small clove garlic, minced, or ⅛ teaspoon garlic powder
¼ cup plus 1 tablespoon shredded fat-free mozzarella cheese
1 pound firm ripe tomatoes, thinly sliced
⅓ cup shredded fresh basil
2 tablespoons grated Parmesan cheese
freshly ground pepper to taste

Preheat the oven to 450°F.

Place the pizza shell on a cookie sheet or pizza stone. Lightly coat the shell with cooking spray. Sprinkle with the scallions and garlic. Top with ¼ cup of the mozzarella cheese. Place the tomatoes in concentric circles covering the pizza, then sprinkle with the basil. Lightly coat with cooking spray. Top with the Parmesan cheese and the remaining mozzarella cheese. Bake until the tomatoes and cheeses just begin to brown and the crust is crisp, about 15 to 18 minutes.

Makes 4 servings.

PER SERVING: 252 calories (21% calories from fat), 6 g total fat (2 g saturated fat), 13 g protein, 36 g carbohydrates, 2 g dietary fiber, 6 mg cholesterol, 578 mg sodium

JOSLIN EXCHANGES: 1 very low fat protein, 2 carbohydrate (2 bread/starch), 1 vegetable, 1 fat

{ Fish and Seafood }

Spicy Grilled Halibut Fillets with Pineapple

Marinating the halibut in pineapple juice with a bit of cumin subtly perks up its mild, sweet flavor. The halibut is deliciously meaty with a medium-firm flesh that shouldn't be cooked dry. Serve this fish with curried couscous prepared from a boxed mix from your market.

1 10-ounce can pineapple slices packed in natural juice
1 clove garlic, minced, or ⅛ teaspoon garlic powder
1 ¾-inch piece fresh ginger, peeled and minced
½ teaspoon ground cumin
⅛ teaspoon crushed red pepper flakes (optional)
2 5-ounce halibut steaks, cut 1 inch thick

Light a gas or charcoal grill, or preheat the broiler.

Drain the pineapple slices and place the juice in a glass baking dish large enough to hold the halibut in a single layer. Combine the juice with the garlic, ginger, cumin, and red pepper flakes (if using). Lay the halibut in the juice mixture and turn once to coat evenly. Set the fish aside to marinate (no more than 30 minutes) while you prepare the rest of the meal.

About 10 minutes before you're ready to eat, grill the halibut 4 to 6 inches from the heat source for 5 minutes, brushing the fish once with the marinade. Turn the halibut and add the pineapple slices to the grill. Continue to cook for another 5 minutes, turning the pineapple once and brushing both the halibut and the pineapple with the marinade.

Place the pineapple slices on top of the halibut and serve immediately.

Makes 2 servings.

PER SERVING: 247 calories (13% calories from fat), 3 g total fat (0.5 g saturated fat), 30 g protein, 23 g carbohydrates, 1 g dietary fiber, 45 mg cholesterol, 79 mg sodium

JOSLIN EXCHANGES: 4 very low fat protein, 1½ carbohydrate (1½ fruit)

How to Buy and Store Fish

Fish is very perishable, so it is important that you know how to buy and store it. Get to know your fishmonger or the person who is behind the fish counter at your supermarket. Shop where the fish is fresh and nicely displayed. Fresh fish does not have a strong odor. If the fish counter has a "fishy" smell, it's likely that the display ice needs changing or the fish case needs a good cleaning. Choose something other than fish if this is the situation. And if the problem persists, talk with the store manager. A good display includes whole fish partially covered by clean ice and fillets in pans surrounded by ice.

If you're buying a whole fish, check that the eyes are bright, clear, and bulging. The fish should have vivid color with no blemishes or skin tears. When you are buying fillets or steaks, look for moist flesh with a translucent sheen. Never buy fillets that have begun to curl—a sure sign that it has been stored too long. Do not buy breaded frozen fish, because you pay exorbitant sums for bread crumbs with very little fish.

Caring for Fresh Fish at Home

Take your fish home promptly and give it a bath in five parts of cool water mixed with one part of lemon juice. (This will kill any bacteria that might have come home with you.) Pat the fish dry with paper towels; wrap in plastic wrap and then aluminum foil. Store in the coldest part of your refrigerator and cook it the same day.

Always wash your hands after handling raw fish. To avoid possible cross-contamination, wash all surfaces and utensils that the fish has touched in hot water with detergent.

Lean fish can be frozen for about two months; oily fish will freeze well for only one month. Commercial flash-frozen fish can remain in the freezer for about three months. You can flash-freeze fresh fish by wetting the fillets and then wrapping them in aluminum foil and freezing solid.

Broiled Cod with Warm Corn and Sweet Onion Relish

In the late spring, when fresh corn begins to appear in the market, this makes a wonderful dinner. Serve the fish on mixed greens or with grilled mushrooms and asparagus. The sweet and sour relish is a good flavor contrast to the mild fish. Another time, serve the corn relish with other grilled meats and poultry.

Warm corn and sweet onion relish:

olive oil cooking spray
½ cup chopped sweet onion, such as Vidalia, Maui, Walla Walla, or Texas
       SuperSweet 1015
1 medium ear fresh corn, kernels cut off the cob
1½ tablespoons white wine vinegar
¼ to ½ teaspoon dry mustard to taste
¼ teaspoon salt (optional)
freshly ground pepper to taste
½ packet sugar substitute (optional)

8 ounces cod fillets

Preheat the broiler.

Lightly coat a nonstick sauté pan with cooking spray and sauté the onion over medium-high heat, stirring frequently, until the onion begins to brown, about 3 to 4 minutes. Add the corn and stir the vegetables for 2 minutes. Lower the heat to medium and add the vinegar, mustard, salt (if using), and pepper. Cook, stirring, for another minute. Remove from the heat and add the sugar substitute (if using).

Lightly coat the cod with cooking spray and broil, 4 to 6 inches from the heat source, until browned and opaque. The total cooking time should be 10 minutes per inch of thickness of the fish.

Divide the cod between 2 plates and place half of the relish down the middle of each piece.

Makes 2 servings.

PER SERVING: 156 calories (9% calories from fat), 2 g total fat (0.2 g saturated fat), 22 g protein, 14 g carbohydrates, 2 g dietary fiber, 49 mg cholesterol, 69 mg sodium

JOSLIN EXCHANGES: 3 very low fat protein, 1 carbohydrate (1 bread/starch)

Swordfish Kebabs

Serve these kebabs over an aromatic long-grain rice such as basmati rice or nuttier-flavored brown rice to which you have added a tablespoon of grated orange zest. This recipe can be doubled or tripled easily to serve company.

Marinade:

½ cup fresh orange juice
1 teaspoon olive oil
1 tablespoon minced fresh tarragon leaves or 1 teaspoon crushed dried
2 cloves garlic, minced, or ¼ teaspoon garlic powder

olive oil cooking spray
8 ounces swordfish, skin removed, cut into 8 cubes
1 10-ounce navel orange, peeled, halved, and cut into 8 pieces
1 medium red onion, cut into 1½-inch squares
1 small red or yellow bell pepper, cut into 1½-inch squares
6 small button mushrooms, stems trimmed

Light a charcoal or gas grill, or preheat the broiler.

To prepare the marinade: In a large bowl, whisk together the orange juice, olive oil, tarragon, and garlic. Add the swordfish cubes and stir gently. Set aside to marinate at room temperature while you prepare the vegetables.

Lightly coat the broiler pan with cooking spray to prevent sticking. Alternate the fruit, vegetables, and swordfish on skewers. Brush with the marinade and place on the grill or under the broiler. Grill or broil for 3 minutes per side, turning once and brushing with marinade. Serve immediately.

Makes 2 servings.

PER SERVING: 312 calories (17% calories from fat), 6 g total fat (1.7 g saturated fat), 27 g protein, 36 g carbohydrates, 6 g dietary fiber, 44 mg cholesterol, 110 mg sodium

JOSLIN EXCHANGES: 3 very low fat protein, 2 carbohydrate (2 fruit), 2 vegetable

Caesar Salad with Grilled Tuna

According to the National Restaurant Association, Caesar salad is the number one salad of the nation. Unfortunately, it's very high in fat and sodium. This recipe uses cubes of grilled tuna in place of fat-laden croutons and an authentic-tasting Caesar-style dressing that is lower in fat and higher in flavor.

8 ounces tuna fillet, skin removed
olive oil cooking spray
⅛ teaspoon garlic powder
freshly ground pepper to taste
4 cups torn, bite-sized pieces of Romaine lettuce, washed, dried, and crisped

Dressing:

1½ tablespoons fresh lemon juice
1 tablespoon olive oil
1 tablespoon water
¼ teaspoon Worcestershire sauce
½ teaspoon Dijon mustard
1 clove garlic, minced, or ⅛ teaspoon garlic powder
¼ teaspoon anchovy paste
2 tablespoons egg substitute
freshly ground pepper to taste

1 tablespoon grated Parmesan cheese

Start a charcoal or gas grill, or preheat the broiler.

Lightly coat the tuna with cooking spray. Season with garlic powder and pepper. Grill or broil over medium heat for 3 to 4 minutes per side, turning once. Transfer the tuna to a cutting board and let rest for 3 minutes before cutting into 1½-inch cubes.

Place the lettuce in a salad bowl.

To make the dressing: In a small bowl, whisk together the dressing ingredients until smooth and creamy. Pour over the lettuce and toss lightly.

Divide the salad between 2 dinner plates. Top with the cubed tuna and sprinkle with the cheese. Serve immediately.

Makes 2 servings.

PER SERVING: 278 calories (45% calories from fat), 14 g total fat (3.1 g saturated fat), 32 g protein, 5 g carbohydrates, 2 g dietary fiber, 46 mg cholesterol, 227 mg sodium

JOSLIN EXCHANGES: 4½ very low fat protein, 2 fat

Barbecued Clams and Mussels

If you live where you can get fresh clams and mussels, this will become one of your favorite grilling recipes. Have a mixed green salad and a bowl of Dilled Rice with Baby Peas (page 184) chilling as a second salad to serve with the barbecued bivalves as they come off the grill. ❡ The sauce is reminiscent of chimichurri sauce, revered by Argentinean cowboys. Another time you can use the sauce with grilled chicken or pork.

Tomato barbecue sauce:

¼ cup dry white wine or water
¼ cup minced red onion
1 clove garlic, minced
2 firm ripe plum tomatoes, minced
3 tablespoons minced fresh basil or flat-leaf parsley
1 red jalapeño chile, seeded and minced
1 tablespoon sherry vinegar

6 cherrystone clams, well scrubbed
16 mussels, well scrubbed

Start a charcoal or gas grill.

To make the sauce: Bring the wine, onion, and garlic to a boil in a small pot over medium-high heat. Cook, stirring, for 2 minutes. Remove from the heat and stir in the tomatoes, basil, chile, and vinegar. Set aside.

When ready to cook, place the unopened clams and mussels in a lightly greased grill over very hot coals. Shellfish are done when they open; mussels will take 1 to 2 minutes, and clams about 3 minutes. Snap off the top side of each bivalve and discard, leaving the clam or mussel in the bottom shell. Spoon a bit of topping on each clam and mussel, and heat on the grill until bubbly, 3 to 5 minutes longer. Serve at once.

Makes 2 servings.

PER SERVING:210 calories (16% calories from fat), 4 g total fat (0.6 g saturated fat), 24 g protein, 12 g carbohydrates, 1 g dietary fiber, 56 mg cholesterol, 278 mg sodium

JOSLIN EXCHANGES: 3 very low fat protein, ½ carbohydrate (½ bread/starch), 1 vegetable

The Many Ways to Use Lemons

We use so many lemons in our cooking that we keep a bowl of them sitting on the kitchen counter. This keeps them handy to use, and storing lemons at room temperature actually increases the juice yield. When selecting lemons, choose ones that feel heavy for their size (the heavier, the juicier) with smooth, unblemished skins and no green areas.

Lemon zest, the yellow part of the peel, is loaded with aromatic oils. Use a zester to scrape away the flavorful peel, leaving the bitter white pith behind. You can use the fine threads made by the zester or mince them further. Lemon zest is a welcome addition to pepper when seasoning meats, fish, poultry, and vegetables. Try both the zest and the juice on fresh melon and fruit salad. Lemon juice will keep cut apples, peaches, pears, and avocados from turning brown. Adding lemon zest and juice to fruit pies, tarts, and crisps intensifies the fruit flavor. Fresh salad greens benefit from a simple dressing of lemon juice and herbs. Many vegetables take on a whole new taste with a sprinkle of lemon zest and a squeeze of lemon juice.

At room temperature, lemons will keep for two weeks. Refrigerated lemons will keep for up to six weeks. Freshly squeezed juice can be frozen for up to four months.

Broiled Sole with Lemon, Tomato, and Capers

This is a really easy dish. The fish cooks in about 6 minutes, so have the rest of the meal ready.

> 2 4-ounce sole fillets
> lemon pepper seasoning to taste
> 1 small, firm, ripe tomato, finely diced
> 1 teaspoon capers, rinsed and well drained
> ¼ teaspoon crushed dried thyme
> ¼ teaspoon garlic powder
> ½ tablespoon fresh lemon juice
> 4 thin slices of lemon for garnish (optional)

Preheat the broiler.

Rinse the fillets and pat dry with paper towels. Sprinkle to taste with lemon pepper seasoning. Place the fish in a single layer in a small baking dish.

In a small bowl, combine the remaining ingredients except the lemon slices. Spoon the mixture onto the fillets, dividing equally and spreading the mixture out slightly. Broil 4 inches from the heat source, without turning the fish, for 5 to 6 minutes, until the fish flakes easily with a fork. Garnish each serving with 2 lemon slices if desired and serve at once.

Makes 2 servings.

PER SERVING: 141 calories (12% calories from fat), 2 g total fat (0.4 g saturated fat), 27 g protein, 3 g carbohydrates, 1 g dietary fiber, 68 mg cholesterol, 172 mg sodium

JOSLIN EXCHANGES: 4 very low fat protein

Grilled Swordfish with Tomato Basil Relish

We usually serve this savory fish on top of a bed of Spinach with Garbanzo Beans (page 190). You can also use the herb rub on boneless, skinless chicken breasts before grilling.

Tomato Basil Relish:

½ tablespoon Dijon mustard
3 tablespoons lemon juice
1 tablespoon balsamic vinegar
1 teaspoon olive oil
1 medium tomato, peeled, seeded, and chopped
1 shallot, minced, or 1 tablespoon minced red onion
2 tablespoons chopped fresh basil

Herb rub:

¼ teaspoon crushed dried basil
¼ teaspoon ground cumin
¼ teaspoon crushed dried oregano
¼ teaspoon crushed dried thyme
⅛ teaspoon freshly ground pepper

2 5-ounce swordfish steaks, cut about 1 inch thick

Start a charcoal or gas grill, or preheat the broiler.

To make the relish: In a small bowl, combine the mustard, lemon juice, and vinegar. Whisk in the oil. Stir in the tomato, shallot, and basil. Transfer the relish to a serving bowl and let stand at room temperature until the swordfish is grilled.

In a small bowl, combine the herb rub ingredients.

Rinse the swordfish and pat dry with paper towels. Rub the herb mixture on both sides of the swordfish. Let stand at room temperature for 5 minutes.

Grill the fish 4 to 6 inches over medium-hot coals or other heat source, for 7 to 10 minutes, turning once. Serve the swordfish with the prepared relish.

Makes 2 servings.

PER SERVING: 236 calories (33% calories from fat), 9 g total fat (1.9 g saturated fat), 29 g protein, 10 g carbohydrates, 1 g dietary fiber, 55 mg cholesterol, 231 mg sodium

JOSLIN EXCHANGES: 4 very low fat protein, 1 vegetable

Baked Salmon with Dill on Steamed Cabbage

This simple preparation allows the sweet flavor of the salmon to come through—with just a bit of "bite" from the mustard. The salmon is served on a bed of lemony steamed cabbage that complements the fish perfectly.

Salmon:

2 5-ounce skinless salmon fillets, roughly the same thickness
1 shallot, minced, or 1 tablespoon minced red onion
2 tablespoons chopped fresh dill or 2 teaspoons dried dill weed
1 tablespoon country-style Dijon mustard
1 tablespoon fresh lemon juice
½ teaspoon canola oil
⅛ teaspoon crushed red pepper flakes
freshly ground pepper to taste

Lemon cabbage:

½ of a 1-pound package (about 2 cups) shredded cabbage
2 teaspoons reduced-fat margarine
1 tablespoon fresh lemon juice
¼ teaspoon salt (optional)
freshly ground pepper to taste

Preheat the oven to 450°F.

Place the fillets in a shallow baking dish, flesh side up (not the side that originally had the skin). In a small bowl, combine the shallot, dill, mustard, lemon juice, canola oil, red pepper flakes, and pepper. Using the back of a spoon, spread the mixture evenly on top of the fillets.

Bake for 8 to 10 minutes, until the salmon flakes easily when tested with a fork.

Meanwhile, place the cabbage in the top of a steamer or in a colander set in a large pot filled with 2 inches of boiling water. Cover and steam for 7 to 10 minutes, until the cabbage is crisp-cooked. Do not overcook.

In a glass measuring cup, combine the margarine, lemon juice, salt (if using), and pepper. Microwave on HIGH for 25 to 30 seconds, until the margarine is melted and the liquid is hot. Transfer the cabbage to a bowl and pour on the lemon-margarine mixture. Toss lightly to coat evenly.

To serve, divide the cabbage between 2 serving plates and top with the salmon. Serve at once.

Makes 2 servings.

PER SERVING: 306 calories (49% calories from fat), 17 g total fat (2.8 g saturated fat), 32 g protein, 7 g carbohydrates, 2 g dietary fiber, 88 mg cholesterol, 315 mg sodium

JOSLIN EXCHANGES: 4½ low fat protein, 1 vegetable

Salmon Baked in Foil with Vegetables

This is a particularly lovely way to cook salmon. When the puffy package is opened at the table, revealing a perfectly cooked piece of salmon ringed with tender vegetables, you'll wish you had invited company for dinner.

2 4-ounce salmon fillets
3 tablespoons fresh lemon juice
1 teaspoon grated lemon zest
salt (optional)
freshly ground pepper to taste
vegetable cooking spray
2 shallots, minced, or 2 tablespoons minced red onion
1 small yellow summer squash, cut into ½-inch rounds
12 cherry tomatoes, stemmed
3 tablespoons coarsely shredded fresh basil
additional fresh basil for garnish (optional)

Preheat the oven to 400°F.

Rinse the fillets and pat dry with paper towels. Measure and note the height of the salmon at its thickest point (it should be about 1 to 1¼ inches). Place the fillets in a glass dish and season with lemon juice, lemon zest, salt (if using), and pepper. Let marinate at room temperature for 5 minutes.

Cut 2 sheets of heavy-duty aluminum foil about 10 x 16 inches. Lightly coat 1 side of each sheet with cooking spray. Place a fillet in the center of each sheet and spoon on the lemon marinade. Top the fillets with shallots and surround with the summer squash and cherry tomatoes, dividing equally. Sprinkle with the basil.

Fold the foil into rectangular envelopes, crimping all the edges. Place the foil packets on a baking sheet and bake for 10 to 12 minutes, using the Canadian Rule for Cooking Fish (below) or until opaque.

To serve, place a packet on each of 2 dinner plates. At the table, slash an ✕ in each packet and peel back the foil. (Be careful, there will be lots of hot steam.) Garnish with basil if desired.

Makes 2 servings.

PER SERVING: 208 calories (33% calories from fat), 8 g total fat (1.2 g saturated fat), 24 g protein, 11 g carbohydrates, 2 g dietary fiber, 62 mg cholesterol, 62 mg sodium

JOSLIN EXCHANGES: 3 low fat protein, 2 vegetable

Oven-Fried Catfish

Catfish is extremely popular where we live, but it's nothing like the muddy-tasting catfish that we fished for in rivers and lakes when we were younger. Today the catfish in our grocery stores and fish markets are farm-raised and have a very mild white flesh. ❡ Since we are watching the fat content, we choose not to have the deep-fried catfish that is served in countless nearby restaurants, but our "oven-fried" version is mighty tasty. You can use almost any white fillet for this recipe—carp, cod, grouper, haddock, orange roughy, ocean perch, pollock, rockfish, red snapper, scrod, or sea bass. Adjust the cooking time accordingly, using the Canadian Rule for Cooking Fish (see below).

The Canadian Rule for Cooking Fish

Determining how long to cook a piece of fish no longer needs to be guesswork. We swear by the rule established by the Canadian Department of Fisheries. It estimates the total cooking time of any fish to be ten minutes for every inch of thickness, measured at the thickest part. This works for fillets, steaks, or whole fish, regardless of the cooking method. Double the time for frozen fish. Try it. It's amazing.

You can also make the fish less spicy by omitting some or all of the herbs and spices except pepper. It won't affect the calories or exchanges.

2 4-ounce catfish fillets
¾ cup skim milk
½ cup yellow cornmeal for dredging
½ teaspoon freshly ground pepper, or to taste
¼ teaspoon chili powder
¼ teaspoon crushed dried thyme
⅛ teaspoon ground cumin
⅛ teaspoon cayenne pepper
salt (optional)
1½ tablespoons reduced-fat margarine, melted
2 lemon wedges (optional)

Soak the fillets in milk while you preheat the oven to its highest temperature, short of broiling.

In a shallow dish, mix the cornmeal with the pepper, chili powder, thyme, cumin, cayenne pepper, and salt (if using). Drain the fillets and dredge them in the cornmeal mixture, patting them to make sure the mixture adheres to both sides.

Drizzle half of the margarine in the bottom of a small baking pan just large enough to hold the 2 fillets in a single layer. Drizzle with the remaining margarine and bake near the top of the oven for about 8 minutes, until the catfish flesh is opaque and tender.

Serve at once with lemon wedges to squeeze over the fish if desired.

Makes 2 servings.

PER SERVING: 240 calories (34% calories from fat), 9 g total fat (2 g saturated fat), 21 g protein, 18 g carbohydrates, 2 g dietary fiber, 66 mg cholesterol, 159 mg sodium

JOSLIN EXCHANGES: 3 very low fat protein, 1 carbohydrate (1 bread/starch), 1 fat

Baked Stuffed Trout

Most supermarkets sell small boned and butterflied rainbow brook trout with the head and tail intact. These small fish are perfect for stuffing and baking. The baked fish can be served whole or cut into medallions. ℈ Served this way with the thyme crème fraîche sauce, the trout is a lightened version of a dish we enjoyed several times at the famous Montrachet French restaurant in New York City.

2 8-ounce rainbow brook trout, butterflied and boned, with heads and tails intact
kosher salt (optional)
freshly ground pepper to taste
butter-flavored cooking spray
2 medium leeks (white part plus 1 inch of green), well rinsed, cut in half lengthwise,
    and thinly sliced
1 clove garlic, thinly sliced
3 tablespoons fat-free reduced-sodium canned chicken broth
½ teaspoon fresh thyme leaves or ⅛ teaspoon crushed dried

Thyme crème fraîche sauce:

⅓ cup Crème Fraîche (page 224) or fat-free sour cream
1 tablespoon minced parsley
½ teaspoon fresh thyme leaves or ⅛ teaspoon crushed dried
⅛ teaspoon freshly ground pepper

Preheat the oven to 450°F.

Rinse the trout and pat dry with paper towels. Open the trout flat and lightly sprinkle the cavity with kosher salt (if using) and pepper.

Lightly coat a small nonstick skillet with cooking spray. Add the leeks and garlic, and sauté over low heat until the leeks begin to wilt, about 4 minutes. Add the chicken broth and thyme leaves. Raise the heat to medium and cook, stirring, until the leeks are tender and the liquid is almost gone (less than a teaspoon remaining).

Stuff the trout cavities with the leek mixture and close the trout over the stuffing. Place the stuffed trout in a shallow baking dish and bake, without turning, for about 15 minutes, until the flesh flakes easily when prodded with a fork.

Meanwhile, in a small bowl, combine the crème fraîche, parsley, thyme, and pepper. When the trout are done, remove the heads and tails with a sharp knife and discard. Serve the stuffed trout whole or slice each into 3 medallions. Arrange on 2 plates and pass the sauce separately to spoon over the fish.

Makes 2 servings.

PER SERVING: 253 calories (32% calories from fat), 9 g total fat (2.8 g saturated fat), 35 g protein, 6 g carbohydrates, <1 g dietary fiber, 101 mg cholesterol, 123 mg sodium

JOSLIN EXCHANGES: 4 very low fat protein, ½ carbohydrate (½ nonfat milk)

Orange Roughy Baked in Foil

Baking fish in foil or parchment paper allows the fish to steam gently in its own juices, keeping it moist. The trick to a perfect steamed fish is to be sure to close the seams securely to prevent leaks. ❡ In this recipe we add orange to the fish to brighten its taste. The very thin slices of orange will cook with the fish, so you can eat the slices, rind and all.

8 ounces orange roughy fillets
2 scallions (white part plus 1 inch of green), cut in half lengthwise
6 thin asparagus spears, woody ends removed
4 very thin slices of an unpeeled navel orange
¼ teaspoon ground ginger
⅛ teaspoon garlic powder
freshly ground pepper to taste
butter-flavored cooking spray
1 tablespoon fresh orange juice

Preheat the oven to 425°F. Cut 2 pieces of aluminum foil approximately 12 x 8 inches (or larger if your fillets are bigger; you'll need about 2½ times the width of the fillet).

Place a fillet in the middle of each piece of foil. Top with the scallions, asparagus, and orange slices. Sprinkle with the ginger, garlic powder, and pepper. Lightly coat the fish with cooking spray. Drizzle ½ tablespoon of orange juice on each fillet. Carefully close the foil and crimp the edges. Transfer the packets to a baking sheet and bake for 8 to 10 minutes, depending on the thickness of the fish.

To serve, place the packets on serving plates. Break open and serve immediately.

Makes 2 servings.

PER SERVING: 120 calories (9% calories from fat), 1 g total fat (trace saturated fat), 22 g protein, 4 g carbohydrates, <1 g dietary fiber, 29 mg cholesterol, 94 mg sodium

JOSLIN EXCHANGES: 3 very low fat protein

Steamed Flounder with Hot Balsamic Sauce

This Chinese method of cooking gives delicate white fish a marvelous flavor. A Chinese steamer is ideal, but if you don't have one, you can improvise by using a wire rack (one you'd use for cooling cakes) that is large enough to hold the fillets in a single layer and that extends just beyond the sides of the skillet. Lay a double sheet of heavy-duty aluminum foil over the rack, folding the edges back several times to form a ridge around the fish. Cut several slashes in the foil to allow the juices to escape. Place the rack over a large skillet filled with 1 inch of water. Cover the fish with more foil or a large lid, and steam until done. ❡ The recipe calls for flounder, but you can also use fillet of sole, orange roughy, or tilapia. The fish takes only a few minutes, so have the rest of the meal partially done or ready to eat.

⅔ pound flounder fillets
olive oil cooking spray
2 tablespoons balsamic vinegar
1½ tablespoons reduced-sodium soy sauce
1 teaspoon olive oil
1 bunch scallions with some tops, thinly sliced

Rinse the fillets and pat dry with paper towels. Place in a Chinese steamer or a devised steamer as described above. Steam for 8 to 10 minutes, depending on the thickness of the fillets, until the fish flakes easily with a fork.

Meanwhile, lightly coat a small nonstick skillet with cooking spray. When the fish is done, transfer to a heated serving platter. Mix together the vinegar and soy sauce. Add the olive oil to the skillet and place over high heat. When the oil is smoking, add the vinegar–soy sauce mixture, then immediately remove the skillet from the stove. Pour the sauce over fish and sprinkle with the scallions. Serve at once.

Makes 2 servings.

PER SERVING: 194 calories (20% calories from fat), 4 g total fat (0.7 g saturated fat), 30 g protein, 7 g carbohydrates, 0 dietary fiber, 72 mg cholesterol, 506 mg sodium

JOSLIN EXCHANGES: 4 very low fat protein, ½ carbohydrate (½ bread/starch)

Scallops with Stewed Tomatoes and Okra

We love stewed tomatoes, and this recipe is not at all like the canned variety. Try stewed tomatoes over pasta or rice, or as a filling for an omelet. It's also good as a condiment for an open-faced grilled reduced-fat cheese sandwich. ❡ Here we've put our stewed tomatoes together with fresh sea scallops and okra for a lovely Creole dish that cooks in minutes. Serve this over steamed white rice.

Stewed tomatoes:

1 14½-ounce can no-salt-added diced tomatoes
¼ cup water
1 tablespoon frozen chopped onion
1 small clove garlic, minced
¼ cup chopped celery
¾ teaspoon brown sugar
¼ to ½ teaspoon curry powder, or to taste
⅛ teaspoon paprika
freshly ground pepper to taste
½ pound sea scallops
1 cup frozen chopped okra

To make the stewed tomatoes: Place the tomatoes, water, onion, garlic, and celery in a large saucepan. Simmer, covered, for 10 minutes. Add the brown sugar, curry powder, paprika, and pepper. Simmer, uncovered, another 2 to 3 minutes.

Add the scallops and okra. Return to a simmer. Stir and cook for 3 to 4 minutes, until the scallops are cooked through and the okra is tender. Serve immediately.

Makes 2 servings.

PER SERVING: 187 calories (8% calories from fat), 2 g total fat (0.2 g saturated fat), 23 g protein, 22 g carbohydrates, 7 g dietary fiber, 37 mg cholesterol, 227 mg sodium

JOSLIN EXCHANGES: 3 very low fat protein, 4 vegetable

Shrimp Fajitas

Fajitas bought in restaurants or in the ready-to-cook section of a supermarket are frequently loaded with fat and sodium. Here's a colorful, easy, delicious, and healthy recipe for fajitas that can be varied as you wish—substituting grilled chicken breast, firm white fish, or flank steak for the shrimp.

olive oil cooking spray
1 medium red onion, cut into ⅓-inch sections and separated into strips
1 large green or yellow bell pepper, cut into ⅓-inch strips
2 cloves garlic, minced, or ¼ teaspoon garlic powder
8 ounces large shrimp (about 25 per pound), peeled and deveined
2 teaspoons Worcestershire sauce
1 tablespoon lemon or lime juice
1 teaspoon ground cumin
freshly ground pepper to taste
1 tablespoon chopped cilantro (optional)
4 7-inch 98% fat-free flour tortillas

Garnishes:

1 cup loosely packed shredded lettuce
½ cup chopped fresh tomatoes
¼ cup mild or hot salsa
¼ cup thinly sliced mushrooms

Lightly coat a large nonstick skillet with cooking spray. Add the onion, bell pepper, and garlic. Sauté over medium-high heat, stirring often, until the vegetables are crisp-cooked, about 3 minutes. Add the shrimp and continue to cook, stirring often, until they turn pink and are just opaque but still moist in the center (cut to test), 3 to 5 minutes. Stir in the Worcestershire sauce, lemon or lime juice, cumin, pepper, and cilantro (if using). Turn the heat to low.

Prepare the tortillas by wrapping them in damp paper towels and heating for 45 seconds to 1 minute in the microwave on HIGH, or follow the directions on the tortilla package.

To serve, spoon the shrimp mixture into the warmed tortillas, dividing equally. Pass the garnishes separately.

Makes 2 servings.

PER SERVING: 362 calories (9% calories from fat), 4 g total fat (0.4 g saturated fat), 30 g protein, 60 g carbohydrates, 13 g dietary fiber, 175 mg cholesterol, 409 mg sodium

JOSLIN EXCHANGES: 3 very low fat protein, 3 carbohydrate (3 bread/starch), 2 vegetable

Low-Fat Open-Faced Tuna Melt

We never tire of this sandwich and frequently find ourselves reaching for a can of tuna when we're eating light. Be sure to buy water-packed tuna, because it has only 17 percent calories from fat, while oil-packed tuna has 80 percent calories from fat.

1 6-ounce can water-packed tuna, well drained
2 tablespoons shredded carrot
2 tablespoons thinly sliced celery
2 tablespoons chopped green apple
1 tablespoon minced red onion
½ tablespoon dill pickle relish
1 hard-cooked egg white, chopped
1 tablespoon plain nonfat yogurt
1 tablespoon reduced-calorie mayonnaise
2 slices nonfat multigrain bread
2 thin slices ripe tomato
1 ounce fat-free Swiss cheese, thinly sliced

Preheat the broiler.

In a medium bowl, combine the tuna, carrot, celery, apple, onion, relish, and egg white. Add the yogurt and mayonnaise, and mix well.

Place the bread slices on a baking sheet and top each with a tomato slice. Add the tuna mixture, dividing equally. Cover evenly with the cheese. Broil 4 inches from the heat source for 3 to 5 minutes, until the cheese is bubbling and golden brown. Serve immediately.

Makes 2 servings.

PER SERVING: 232 calories (13% calories from fat), 3 g total fat (0.7 g saturated fat), 30 g protein, 20 g carbohydrates, 2 g dietary fiber, 28 mg cholesterol, 732 mg sodium

JOSLIN EXCHANGES: 4 very low fat protein, 1 carbohydrate (1 bread/starch)

Baked Crab Cakes with Roasted Red Pepper Sauce

Crab cakes are always a special treat, but they're usually fried in olive oil. These are baked to reduce fat grams and served with an intriguing roasted red pepper sauce. Don't be intimidated by the list of ingredients. The crab cakes go together in minutes, the sauce is a snap, and the whole dish is well worth the effort.

Crab cakes:

vegetable cooking spray
8 ounces fresh lump crabmeat
1 large egg white
2 tablespoons finely minced celery
1 tablespoon minced red onion
¼ fresh jalapeño chile pepper, minced
½ tablespoon reduced-calorie mayonnaise
⅛ teaspoon dry mustard
⅛ teaspoon freshly ground pepper
dash cayenne pepper
dash hot pepper sauce
½ tablespoon fresh lemon juice
¼ teaspoon Worcestershire sauce
1 tablespoon minced flat-leaf parsley
½ cup unseasoned dry bread crumbs

Roasted red pepper sauce:

½ of a 7-ounce jar roasted red bell peppers, drained
⅓ cup fat-free sour cream
⅛ teaspoon hot pepper sauce
⅛ teaspoon crushed dried thyme

Preheat the oven to 400°F. Lightly coat a nonstick baking sheet with cooking spray.

Rinse the crabmeat in a fine strainer under cold running water, making sure to remove all filaments and shells. Drain well.

In a medium bowl, combine the remaining crab cake ingredients, except ¼ cup of bread crumbs. Stir in the well-drained crabmeat. Form the mixture into 4 patties, roll them in the reserved bread crumbs, and place on the prepared baking sheet.

To prepare the sauce: Place the roasted bell peppers, sour cream, hot pepper sauce, and thyme in a food processor or blender. Puree until smooth. Transfer the mixture to a small saucepan and heat slowly on the stove while the crab cakes are baking. Do not let the sauce come to a boil or it will separate. (It is best when only slightly warm.)

Lightly coat the crab cakes with the cooking spray. Bake on the bottom rack of the oven for 5 minutes per side, turning once, until the crab cakes are nicely browned.

To serve, spoon the warm sauce onto 2 plates, making a "puddle" in the middle. Top with the crab cakes and serve immediately.

Makes 2 servings.

PER SERVING: 298 calories (13% calories from fat), 4 g total fat (0.7 g saturated fat), 30 g protein, 31 g carbohydrates, 1 g dietary fiber, 114 mg cholesterol, 806 mg sodium

JOSLIN EXCHANGES: 3 very low fat protein, 2 carbohydrate (2 bread/starch)

Cold Poached Salmon with Cucumber Sauce

On a hot summer night, nothing is better than a cold seafood supper—especially cold salmon with a refreshing cucumber sauce made of cooling yogurt. Make the salmon and sauce early in the day (or the night before) so they have plenty of time to chill in the refrigerator. ❡ Serve the salmon with cold steamed baby carrots, sugar snap peas, and a crusty roll. Go easy with dessert, perhaps a scoop of your favorite flavor of fat-free frozen yogurt or ice cream.

1 quart water
¼ cup dry white wine or additional water
2 tablespoons lemon juice
1 large bay leaf
¼ teaspoon black peppercorns
2 4-ounce salmon steaks, cut 1 inch thick

Cucumber sauce:

⅓ cup plain nonfat yogurt
½ teaspoon minced garlic
¼ cup coarsely grated peeled cucumber
1 scallion (white part plus 1 inch of green), minced
½ tablespoon minced fresh cilantro
dash salt (optional)
freshly ground pepper to taste
⅛ teaspoon cumin seed
2 sprigs fresh cilantro for garnish (optional)

In a large heavy-bottomed skillet, combine the water, wine, lemon juice, bay leaf, and peppercorns. Cover and bring to a rapid boil over high heat.

Add the salmon steaks, cover, and turn off the heat. Let the salmon sit for about 8 minutes, until still moist-looking but opaque in the thickest part (cut to test). Do not disturb until it is time to test. If not done, cover the skillet again and let stand until it tests done.

Using a slotted pancake turner, transfer the salmon to a plate. Cover tightly with plastic wrap and chill for at least 1 hour or up to 1 day. Discard the poaching liquid.

To make the sauce: In a small bowl, combine all the sauce ingredients except the cilantro. Chill until ready to serve with the salmon.

Arrange the salmon steaks on 2 serving plates, spoon the sauce over each portion, and garnish with a cilantro sprig if desired.

Makes 2 servings.

PER SERVING: 196 calories (36% calories from fat), 7 g total fat (1.2 g saturated fat), 25 g protein, 5 g carbohydrates, <1 g dietary fiber, 63 mg cholesterol, 82 mg sodium

JOSLIN EXCHANGES: 3½ low fat protein

{ Poultry }

Cajun Grilled Chicken on Yellow Rice and Peas

Most supermarkets carry several brands of Cajun spice mixes, usually a blend of black pepper, red pepper, garlic, and thyme. Choose one that doesn't contain salt or MSG and keep it handy for seasoning chicken, turkey, and fish.

2 4-ounce boneless, skinless chicken breast fillets
3 tablespoons fresh lemon juice
½ teaspoon Cajun spice mix
dash hot pepper sauce (optional)
½ cup fat-free reduced-sodium canned chicken broth
½ cup water
¼ cup frozen baby peas
1 cup uncooked instant rice
⅛ teaspoon crushed saffron threads or ground turmeric
½ tablespoon chopped pimiento (optional), well drained

Start a charcoal or gas grill, or preheat the broiler.

Rinse the chicken fillets and pat dry with paper towels. Place in a shallow glass baking dish. In a small bowl, combine the lemon juice, Cajun spice mix, and hot pepper sauce (if using). Pour over the chicken and turn once to coat evenly. Let stand at room temperature for 10 minutes.

Remove the chicken from the marinade. Grill or broil the chicken 4 to 6 inches from the medium-hot heat source for 6 to 7 minutes per side, turning once. Chicken is done when opaque throughout (cut to test).

While the chicken is grilling, bring the broth and water to a boil in a small saucepan. Place the peas in a microwave-safe covered dish, and microwave on DE-FROST for 1 minute. When the broth mixture boils, stir in the peas, rice, and saffron. Cover and set aside for 5 minutes. Fluff the rice with a fork and stir in pimiento.

To serve, divide the rice-pea mixture between 2 plates. Top with the grilled chicken and serve at once.

Makes 2 servings.

PER SERVING: 335 calories (5% calories from fat), 2 g total fat (0.7 g saturated fat), 32 g protein, 45 g carbohydrates, 2 g dietary fiber, 66 mg cholesterol, 226 mg sodium

JOSLIN EXCHANGES: 3 very low fat protein, 3 carbohydrate (3 bread/starch)

Grilled Chicken Salad with Summer Salsa Dressing

By the end of June we are watching the farmer's market closely because that's when vine-ripened tomatoes and sweet corn are local and fresh. Here the summer favorites play a double role: They are the basis for a salsa, which then becomes the dressing for the salad. You can buy the baby lettuces for this salad already mixed, washed, and ready to use in convenient packages at most supermarkets. ❧ You can also double the recipe for salsa and use it to stuff a Mexican omelet made with egg substitute.

Summer salsa dressing:

2 medium ears of fresh corn
1 medium, firm, ripe tomato, seeded and chopped
1 clove garlic, minced, or ⅛ teaspoon garlic powder
2 scallions (white part only), thinly sliced
2 tablespoons frozen chopped green pepper
1 to 2 tablespoons chopped cilantro, or to taste
½ teaspoon ground cumin
⅛ teaspoon kosher salt (optional)
freshly ground pepper to taste
1½ tablespoons fresh lemon juice
1 tablespoon olive oil
2 tablespoons water

Grilled Chicken Salad:

8 ounces skinless, boneless chicken breast halves, pounded thin (see page 126)
4 cups mixed baby lettuces, crisped

Start a charcoal or gas grill, or preheat the broiler.

Pull the husks off the corn and remove the silks. (Any stubborn silks can be brushed off with your hand or a soft cloth.) Wrap each ear securely in white paper towels, twisting the ends tightly to seal. Cook in the microwave on HIGH for 4 to 5 minutes, turning each ear once. Cool the corn to the touch. Then, using a sharp knife, cut off the kernels from the cob, 3 or 4 rows at a time. Place the kernels in a bowl and add the tomato, garlic, scallions, green pepper, cilantro, cumin, salt (if using), ground pepper, lemon juice, olive oil, and water. Stir and set aside.

Grill or broil the chicken, 4 to 6 inches from the heat source, for 5 minutes per side, turning once. Place on a carving board and slice the meat against the grain into thin slices.

Divide the lettuces between 2 plates. Arrange the chicken slices in a fan shape on top and surround with the salsa dressing.

Makes 2 servings.

PER SERVING: 328 calories (27% calories from fat), 10 g total fat (1.6 g saturated fat),32 g protein, 31 g carbohydrates, 6 g dietary fiber, 66 mg cholesterol, 109 mg sodium

JOSLIN EXCHANGES: 3½ very low fat protein, 2 carbohydrate (2 bread/starch), 1 vegetable, 1 fat

Safe Handling of Poultry

Poultry from even the best of supermarkets requires special precautions before and after you get it home. At the supermarket, check the expiration date and buy only the freshest poultry. Make it one of the last purchases to go into your cart and take it home immediately.

Once home, remove the chicken or other form of poultry from its wrappings; rinse thoroughly with cold water and pat dry with paper towels. Remove and discard any giblet packages (organ meats are very high in cholesterol and should be eaten only very occasionally). Also remove and discard any visible lumps of fat.

If you aren't cooking the poultry immediately, wrap it loosely in aluminum foil and store in the coldest part of the refrigerator for no more than forty-eight hours. Never let poultry sit at room temperature for more than fifteen minutes.

To avoid possible cross-contamination, wash your hands, cutting knives, and work surfaces with hot soapy water after handling raw poultry. For example, don't handle a piece of raw chicken and then make a tossed salad without a thorough hand washing in between.

To freeze poultry, wrap it airtight in freezer wrap or heavy plastic wrap. Mark the date and weight of the poultry. Freeze solidly and use within three months. Always thaw frozen poultry in the refrigerator—never on the countertop. Do not refreeze uncooked poultry.

Lemon-Peppered Chicken Breasts with Raisins and Sunflower Seeds

Boneless chicken breast halves are quick-cooking and economical, and with the right seasonings, they can turn a simple dish into a special main course. Couscous would be good to serve with the chicken, along with Green Beans with Herbs (page 198).

2 4-ounce skinless, boneless chicken breast halves, pounded thin (see page 126)
¼ teaspoon garlic salt (optional)
¼ teaspoon lemon pepper seasoning
¼ teaspoon crushed dried oregano
⅛ teaspoon crushed red pepper flakes, or to taste
1 tablespoon olive oil
1½ tablespoons balsamic vinegar
2 tablespoons dark raisins
1 tablespoon dry-roasted sunflower seeds
1 tablespoon chopped parsley for garnish (optional)
½ fresh lemon, cut into wedges, for garnish (optional)

Rinse the chicken breast halves and pat dry with paper towels. Start a charcoal or gas grill, or preheat the broiler.

Sprinkle the chicken breasts with garlic salt (if using), lemon pepper, oregano, and red pepper flakes.

Grill the breasts, 4 to 6 inches from the medium-high heat source, for 4 minutes per side, until no longer pink inside (cut to test). Transfer to 2 plates and keep warm.

Meanwhile, in a small pan, bring the olive oil, vinegar, raisins, and sunflower seeds to a full boil over high heat for 30 seconds. Immediately spoon the mixture over the chicken breasts and sprinkle with parsley, if desired. Serve with the lemon wedges, if desired, to squeeze over all.

Makes 2 servings.

PER SERVING: 249 calories (36% calories from fat), 10 g total fat (1.5 g saturated fat), 27 g protein, 12 carbohydrates, <1 g dietary fiber, 66 mg cholesterol, 78 mg sodium

JOSLIN EXCHANGES: 4 very low fat protein, 1 carbohydrate (1 fruit)

Fast and Easy Chicken Breasts

We keep boneless, skinless chicken breast halves, pounded flat, in our freezer for quick, impromptu dinners. Since they are quite thin, there is no need to thaw before cooking, and they cook in about 5 minutes per side on a grill or under a broiler. The pounded breasts can also be poached in the microwave in a covered container with a little water (takes only 5 minutes) or sautéed in a nonstick skillet that has been coated with cooking spray.

To pound chicken breasts, place each breast half between two pieces of plastic wrap and lightly pound with the flat side of a meat pounder to about ½ inch thickness. Remove and discard the plastic wrap. Cook as desired or wrap each pounded half securely in fresh plastic wrap. Package several pounded halves in a self-sealing plastic freezer bag (they'll separate easily while still frozen). Date the package and note the number of pieces. Use within three months.

Chicken Breasts Stuffed with Feta Cheese and Spinach

In this recipe, pounded chicken breasts are rolled up with a feta cheese and fresh spinach stuffing. When they're cooked and sliced, you'll have colorful pinwheels that look as if you went to a lot of work to prepare them—but you didn't.

6 leaves fresh spinach, well rinsed and stems removed
2 4-ounce chicken breast halves, pounded (see above) and thawed, if frozen
3 tablespoons crumbled feta cheese
2 teaspoons fresh lemon juice
freshly ground pepper to taste
3 tablespoons flour for dredging
olive oil cooking spray

Preheat the oven to 400°F.

Cook the spinach leaves in boiling water for 1 minute. Drain and squeeze out all the moisture. Place the chicken on a work surface with the wide side toward you. Arrange 3 spinach leaves over each chicken breast, distributing them evenly and leaving a ½-inch border at the top edge. Sprinkle with half of the feta cheese and half of the lemon juice. Season with pepper. Starting at the bottom wide edge, roll the chicken breast into a tight cylinder. Pin it closed with toothpicks. Fill, roll, and close the second breast.

Dredge each rolled chicken breast in the flour, shaking off the excess. Lightly coat a nonstick skillet that has an ovenproof handle with cooking spray. Place over medium-high heat and add the chicken breasts. Sauté until the chicken is lightly browned on all sides, about 5 minutes. Place the skillet with the chicken breasts in the oven and bake until done, 15 to 20 minutes.

Transfer the chicken to a cutting board and remove the toothpicks. Cut each breast crosswise into ½-inch slices. Fan the slices out on 2 plates. Serve at once.

Makes 2 servings.

PER SERVING: 191 calories (19% calories from fat), 4 g total fat (2.3 g saturated fat), 30 g protein, 8 g carbohydrates, 1 g dietary fiber, 75 mg cholesterol, 212 mg sodium

JOSLIN EXCHANGES: 4 very low fat protein, ½ carbohydrate (½ bread/starch)

Ten Ways to Dress Up Grilled or Broiled Chicken Breasts

1. Marinate the chicken in lime juice and cumin before cooking. Serve with salsa.

2. Top the cooked chicken with a combination of sliced or whole sautéed mushrooms and thyme.

3. Top the cooked chicken with caramelized (cooked until golden) onion rings.

4. Serve the cooked chicken with a homemade fresh fruit relish.

5. Top the cooked chicken with fresh raspberries that have been heated in a little balsamic vinegar.

6. Top the cooked chicken with grilled fresh fruit slices.

7. Reduce dry white wine by half and add garlic, lemon juice, and pepper. Pour over the cooked chicken.

8. Make a paste of coarse mustard, garlic, and onion. Spread the mixture over the chicken when you turn to cook the second side.

9. Make a quick tomato sauce with a chopped fresh tomato, minced garlic, and minced fresh basil. Spoon over the cooked chicken.

10. Top the cooked chicken with sauce made from minced fresh ginger, minced garlic, some dry sherry, and a little reduced-sodium soy sauce.

Check the Joslin Exchanges (page 249) to determine how each will affect your exchanges.

Baked Chicken Quesadillas

Filled with nonfat refried beans and shredded chicken, these quesadillas are hearty and filling. Pair them with summer fruit salad (page 205) for a quick supper. ℐ If your market doesn't carry nonfat refried beans, mash drained canned pinto beans with a little red wine vinegar.

vegetable cooking spray
¼ cup fat-free canned refried beans
½ teaspoon chili powder
2 7-inch 98% fat-free flour tortillas
½ cup shredded cooked chicken
½ cup shredded reduced-fat Monterey Jack or sharp cheddar cheese
1 small, firm, ripe plum tomato, chopped
2 tablespoons minced red onion
2 tablespoons minced fresh cilantro
*½ cup Fresh Tomato Salsa (page 97) or 2 tablespoons bottled salsa (this adds 153 mg
     sodium)*

Preheat the oven to 500°F. Lightly coat a baking sheet with cooking spray.

In a small bowl, mix the refried beans and chili powder. Lightly brush both sides of each tortilla with water. Spread half of the refried beans over half of each tortilla. Cover the beans evenly on each tortilla with half of the chicken, cheese, tomato, onion, and cilantro. Fold over the other half of each tortilla to cover the filling.

Set the quesadillas on the prepared baking sheet at least 3 inches apart. Bake until crisp and golden, about 7 minutes. Transfer to 2 serving plates. Cut into wedges and serve with salsa.

Makes 2 servings.

PER SERVING: 268 calories (21% calories from fat), 6 g total fat (3.9 g saturated fat), 24 g protein, 33 g carbohydrates, 7 g dietary fiber, 44 mg cholesterol, 670 mg sodium

JOSLIN EXCHANGES: 2½ low fat protein, 2 carbohydrate (2 bread/starch)

Chicken Curry

Here is a chicken curry that is pungent and hot. We use an imported hot Indian curry powder and gain additional heat from garlic and fresh ginger. If you like your food less spicy, use half of the spice mix called for and reduce the fresh ginger to 1 teaspoon (or ¼ teaspoon of ground ginger). You can add more spice mix as needed to get the heat intensity you like. ❡ Serve the curry with steamed basmati rice that has been cooked with a bit of shredded carrot, and offer the Cucumber Sauce (page 120) for a nice cooling condiment. End the meal with a piece of fresh mango or melon.

8 ounces boneless, skinless chicken breast fillets
salt (optional)
freshly ground pepper to taste
olive oil cooking spray
½ cup frozen chopped onion
1 clove garlic, minced, or ⅛ teaspoon garlic powder
½ tablespoon finely minced fresh ginger or ½ teaspoon ground ginger
½ tablespoon hot Indian curry powder
⅛ teaspoon cayenne pepper
dash ground cinnamon
dash ground cloves
dash ground coriander
1 cup no-salt-added diced canned tomatoes
⅓ cup fat-free reduced-sodium canned chicken broth
½ tablespoon golden raisins for garnish (optional)

Rinse the chicken breast fillets and pat dry with paper towels. Season with salt (if using) and pepper.

Lightly coat a nonstick sauté pan with cooking spray. Place over medium-high heat and add the chicken breasts. Sauté for 4 to 5 minutes per side, until nicely browned. Transfer the chicken to a plate and keep warm.

Add the onion and garlic to the pan. Turn the heat to low and sauté until the onion wilts, about 4 minutes. Stir in the ginger and cook another minute. In a small bowl, mix together the curry powder, cayenne pepper, cinnamon, cloves, coriander, and pepper. Stir the spices into the pan (start with 1 teaspoon of this mixture for a milder curry). Stir in the tomatoes and broth. Return the chicken pieces to the pan, cover, and simmer for 13 to 15 minutes, until the chicken is tender and cooked through (cut to test).

To serve, transfer the chicken pieces to 2 serving plates. Raise the heat to medium-high and cook the sauce for another 1 or 2 minutes, stirring constantly, to thicken. Spoon sauce over the chicken and, if desired, sprinkle on the raisins. Serve at once.

Makes 2 servings.

PER SERVING: 184 calories (9% calories from fat), 2 g total fat (0.4 g saturated fat), 29 g protein, 14 g carbohydrates, 3 g dietary fiber, 66 mg cholesterol, 194 mg sodium

JOSLIN EXCHANGES: 4 very low fat protein, 2 vegetable

Chicken Tacos

These soft tacos are full of Tex-Mex flavor but contain little fat. Serve them with Ji-cama Slaw (page 208) and a combination of seasonal fruit (page 205) for a quick and easy supper.

1 6-ounce boneless, skinless chicken breast
olive oil cooking spray
3 tablespoons minced onion
1 small clove garlic, minced, or ⅛ teaspoon garlic powder
¼ teaspoon chili powder
¼ teaspoon ground cumin
¼ teaspoon crushed dried oregano
dash cayenne pepper
salt (optional)
freshly ground pepper to taste
4 6-inch corn tortillas

Garnishes:

1 cup shredded lettuce
2 tablespoons shredded reduced-fat Monterey Jack cheese
1 tablespoon coarsely chopped fresh cilantro (optional)
½ cup Fresh Tomato Salsa (page 97) or ¼ cup bottled salsa (this adds 308 mg of sodium)
¼ cup fat-free sour cream

Rinse the chicken breast and pat dry with paper towels. Trim off any fat. Mince the chicken breast as finely as possible.

Preheat the oven to 350°F. Lightly coat a nonstick skillet with cooking spray. Add the onion and garlic. Cook over low heat until the onion wilts, about 4 minutes. Add the minced chicken, chili powder, cumin, oregano, cayenne pepper, salt (if using), and pepper. Cook, stirring constantly, until the chicken is cooked through, about 5 minutes.

Wrap the tortillas in aluminum foil and heat in the oven for 5 minutes, until warm and pliable.

To serve, place the hot chicken filling in a small serving bowl. Mix together the lettuce, cheese, and cilantro, if desired and place in a bowl. Put the salsa and sour cream in separate bowls.

To serve, place a heaping tablespoon of the chicken filling on a tortilla. Top with some of the garnishes. Fold in half or roll into a cylinder for eating.

Makes 2 servings.

PER SERVING (WITH FRESH SALSA): 268 calories (13% calories from fat), 4 g total fat (0.2 g saturated fat), 27 g protein, 30 g carbohydrates, 1 g dietary fiber, 54 mg cholesterol, 151 mg sodium

JOSLIN EXCHANGES: 3 very low fat protein, 1½ carbohydrate (1½ bread/starch), 1 vegetable

Yogurt Cinnamon Chicken

This chicken goes well with dried fruit–studded Mediterranean-style rice or couscous. Making a double recipe of the chicken allows for an excellent chicken salad or sandwich the next day.

¼ cup plain nonfat yogurt
1 teaspoon olive oil
2 cloves garlic, minced, or ¼ teaspoon garlic powder
¾ teaspoon minced fresh ginger or ¼ teaspoon dried ginger
½ teaspoon ground cinnamon
¼ teaspoon ground cumin
¼ teaspoon onion powder
1 teaspoon red wine vinegar
¼ teaspoon kosher salt (optional)
freshly ground pepper to taste
1 8-ounce whole skinless, boneless chicken breast, cut in half
olive oil cooking spray

Preheat the broiler.

In a 2-cup measuring cup, whisk together the yogurt, olive oil, garlic, ginger, cinnamon, cumin, onion powder, vinegar, salt (if using), and pepper. Place the chicken breast halves in a shallow nonreactive baking dish. Set aside 1 tablespoon of the yogurt mixture and spoon the remaining mixture over the chicken, turning once to coat evenly. Set aside to marinate for 15 minutes.

Lightly coat a broiler pan with cooking spray. Place the chicken, skin side down, on the broiler pan. Broil 4 inches from the heat source for 10 to 12 minutes, until nicely browned. Turn, baste with the reserved yogurt mixture, and continue to broil until the breasts are done, about 5 minutes.

Makes 2 servings.

PER SERVING: 171 calories (21% calories from fat), 4 g total fat (0.7 g saturated fat), 28 g protein, 5 g carbohydrates, <1 g dietary fiber, 66 mg cholesterol, 98 mg sodium

JOSLIN EXCHANGES: 4 very low fat protein

All-American Turkey Loaves

Serve this with a mixture of sautéed mushrooms and onions, and add mashed potatoes. *Voilà,* you have a comfort meal like those we can all recall from our youth.

vegetable cooking spray
8 ounces very lean ground turkey breast
2 tablespoons quick rolled oats
2 tablespoons frozen chopped onion
1 clove garlic, minced, or ⅛ teaspoon garlic powder
½ teaspoon Dijon mustard
½ teaspoon tomato paste
¼ teaspoon Worcestershire sauce
2 tablespoons egg substitute
⅛ teaspoon crushed dried thyme
⅛ teaspoon crushed dried marjoram
freshly ground pepper to taste
1 small bay leaf, cut in half

Preheat the oven to 425°F. Lightly coat a small shallow baking dish with cooking spray.

Place the turkey in a medium bowl. Add the oats, onion, garlic, mustard, tomato paste, Worcestershire sauce, egg substitute, thyme, marjoram, and pepper. Mix well. Wet your hands before forming the mixture into 2 loaves of equal size.

Place the loaves in the prepared baking dish. Top each loaf with a bay leaf half. Lightly coat the loaves with cooking spray and bake for 20 to 25 minutes. Check after 15 minutes and lower the oven heat to 400°F if the top is browning too quickly. Be sure to remove the bay leaf halves before eating.

Makes 2 servings.

PER SERVING: 157 calories (13% calories from fat), 2 g total fat (0.5 g saturated fat), 30 g protein, 5 g carbohydrates, 1 g dietary fiber, 70 mg cholesterol, 136 mg sodium

JOSLIN EXCHANGES: 4 very low fat protein

Turkey Scaloppine Marsala

Marsala wines are one of Italy's gifts to the world of food. Sweet Marsala is used for desserts, while dry Marsala, called for in this recipe, is splendid for making rich sauces for poultry, meat, and fish. ❡ Most, but not all, of the alcohol is evaporated during the cooking process. If you prefer not to cook with alcohol or your doctor has advised you to avoid alcohol totally, you can substitute an equal amount of low-sodium beef broth, or plain water plus 1 tablespoon of red wine or balsamic vinegar, with good results.

butter-flavored cooking spray
8 ounces turkey tenderloin, cut on the diagonal against the grain into scallops ⅛ inch
     thick, white membrane discarded
1 teaspoon all-purpose flour
4 ounces button mushrooms, sliced
1 tablespoon fresh lemon juice
¼ cup low-sodium canned beef broth
3 tablespoons dry Marsala wine or dry sherry

Lightly coat with cooking spray a nonstick sauté pan that has a cover.

Dust the turkey scallops with the flour and brown over high heat, turning often to ensure even cooking. Add the mushrooms and cook for 2 minutes.

Lower the heat to medium. Add the lemon juice, beef broth, and Marsala. Cover and simmer for 5 minutes. Transfer the turkey to a heated platter and keep warm.

Raise the heat to high and boil the pan drippings, stirring, until the sauce begins to become syrupy. Return the turkey to the pan and turn to coat evenly. Serve immediately.

Makes 2 servings.

PER SERVING: 157 calories (9% calories from fat), 2 g total fat (0.4 g saturated fat), 29 g protein, 5 g carbohydrates, 1 g dietary fiber, 70 mg cholesterol, 71 mg sodium

JOSLIN EXCHANGES: 4 very low fat protein

Spaghetti with Turkey Meatballs and Basil Tomato Sauce

This is a healthy version of an American favorite. Making your own sauce cuts down on the sodium and fat. The results taste fresh and light. Use the leftover sauce the next day with grilled vegetables for another pasta dish.

Basil tomato sauce:

½ cup frozen chopped onion
2 cloves garlic, minced, or ¼ teaspoon garlic powder
1 28-ounce can no-salt-added crushed tomatoes
2 tablespoons chopped fresh basil or 2 teaspoons crushed dried
freshly ground pepper to taste

Meatballs:

8 ounces very lean ground turkey breast
1 tablespoon egg substitute
1 tablespoon cold water
3 tablespoons quick-cooking oats
⅛ teaspoon garlic powder
⅛ teaspoon onion powder
¼ teaspoon salt (optional)
freshly ground pepper to taste

4 ounces dry spaghetti

In a large nonstick saucepan, sauté the onion and garlic over medium heat until the onion is wilted but not browned, about 3 minutes. Add the crushed tomatoes, half of the basil, and the pepper. Bring to a simmer and continue cooking, uncovered, while you make the turkey balls.

In a medium bowl, combine the turkey, egg substitute, water, oats, garlic powder, onion powder, salt (if using), and pepper. Mix well. Form into 6 meatballs and place them gently in the simmering tomato sauce.

Cover the pan, return to a simmer, and cook for 15 minutes. Gently shake the pan every so often to make sure the turkey balls remain covered with sauce and that they cook on all sides. For thicker sauce, uncover for the last few minutes and raise the heat. Stir in the remaining basil.

Meanwhile, prepare the spaghetti according to the package directions. Drain and keep warm. Divide the spaghetti between 2 plates. Top each plate with 3 turkey balls and ¾ cup of sauce. Refrigerate the remaining sauce.

Makes 2 servings with about 1½ cups of sauce left over.

PER SERVING: 423 calories (6% calories from fat), 3 g total fat (0.6 g saturated fat), 39 g protein, 60 g carbohydrates, 10 g dietary fiber, 70 mg cholesterol, 386 mg sodium

JOSLIN EXCHANGES: 4 very low fat protein, 3 carbohydrate (3 bread/starch), 2 vegetable

Turkey Cutlets with Warm Fruit Relish

Similar to chutney, this warm fruit relish captures both sweet and sour flavors and offers a special accent to a simple meal. You can substitute pears for the apples in this relish, but you'll need to double the lemon juice to get the proper balance of sweet to sour.

½ lemon
8 ounces turkey cutlets
⅛ teaspoon garlic powder
⅛ teaspoon onion powder
freshly ground pepper to taste

Warm fruit relish:

butter-flavored cooking spray
2 tablespoons minced sweet white onion
1 6-ounce sweet firm apple such as Golden Delicious, pared and chopped
¼ teaspoon minced garlic
1½ tablespoons malt vinegar
½ teaspoon ground ginger
½ teaspoon ground cinnamon
½ teaspoon grated lemon zest
1 teaspoon lemon juice
½ packet sugar substitute, or to taste

Light a charcoal or gas grill, or preheat the broiler.

Squeeze the lemon over the cutlets. Combine the garlic powder, onion powder, and pepper, and sprinkle on both sides of the turkey. Grill or broil, 4 to 6 inches from the heat source, for 1 to 2 minutes per side, turning once, until the turkey is no longer pink inside (cut to test). Transfer to a serving platter and keep warm.

Prepare the fruit relish: Lightly coat a small nonstick saucepan with cooking spray. Add the onion and apple, and sauté over medium-high heat for 1 minute. Add the garlic, vinegar, ginger, cinnamon, lemon zest, and lemon juice. Lower heat, partially cover, and simmer for 8 minutes, until the apple is soft. Remove from the heat and add the sugar substitute.

Cut the turkey across the grain into thin slices. Divide between 2 plates and top with some of the warm relish.

Makes 2 servings.

PER SERVING: 184 calories (8% calories from fat), 2 g total fat (0.4 g saturated fat), 27 g protein, 17 g carbohydrates, 3 g dietary fiber, 70 mg cholesterol, 62 mg sodium

JOSLIN EXCHANGES: 4 very low fat protein, 1 carbohydrate (1 fruit)

Grilled Turkey Burgers with Pineapple

Serve these delicious burgers with a plate of fresh vegetables (carrot sticks, celery sticks, radishes, cucumber slices, and so forth). Your favorite fruit-flavored nonfat frozen yogurt or nonfat ice cream would be nice for dessert.

Feel free to add mustard and lettuce or alfalfa sprouts to your burger. Either would be considered "a free food." Go easy on the mustard if you are on a sodium-restricted diet.

> *1 egg white*
> *1 tablespoon dry white wine or water*
> *2 tablespoons seasoned dry bread crumbs (see page 91)*
> *⅓ pound very lean ground turkey breast*
> *1 tablespoon minced red onion*
> *⅛ teaspoon salt (optional)*
> *⅛ teaspoon freshly ground pepper*
> *2 slices canned pineapple packed in natural juice*
> *2 sesame hamburger buns, split and toasted*

Start a charcoal or gas grill, or preheat the broiler.

In a small bowl, whisk together the egg white and wine. Stir in the bread crumbs, ground turkey, onion, salt (if using), and pepper. Mix well. Shape into 2 patties of equal size, about ½ inch thick.

Grill or broil, 4 inches from the heat source, for 5 to 6 minutes per side, turning once. When you turn the burgers, add the pineapple slices to the grill. Turn the pineapple after 3 minutes and grill for another 3 minutes. The turkey patties are done if the juices run clear when a knife is inserted in the center.

To serve, place the grilled patties on the toasted buns, topping each with a slice of grilled pineapple. Serve at once.

Makes 2 servings.

PER SERVING: 302 calories (12% calories from fat), 4 g total fat (0.9 g saturated fat), 25 g protein, 40 g carbohydrates, 2 g dietary fiber, 46 mg cholesterol, 434 mg sodium

JOSLIN EXCHANGES: 3 very low fat protein, 2½ carbohydrate (2 bread/starch, ½ fruit)

Jamaican Turkey Patties

Throughout the island of Jamaica, bakeries and street vendors sell spicy meat turnovers, called patties, for light meals and quick snacks. Ground turkey also works well in the filling and has fewer calories and fat grams. For convenience and fewer fat grams, we use refrigerated canned buttermilk biscuits in place of the customary buttery pastry dough. Eat the turnover hot or warm, out of hand or with a fork.

8 ounces extra-lean ground turkey breast
2 small plum tomatoes, finely chopped
¼ cup minced onion
2 tablespoons minced celery
1 fresh jalapeño chile pepper, seeded and minced
1 clove garlic, minced, or ⅛ teaspoon garlic powder
½ teaspoon curry powder
¼ teaspoon ground ginger
¼ teaspoon crushed dried thyme
¼ teaspoon salt (optional)
freshly ground pepper to taste
1 teaspoon cornstarch
1 tablespoon dry sherry or water
¼ cup fat-free reduced-sodium chicken broth
1 6-ounce can refrigerated buttermilk biscuits

Preheat the oven to 400°F.

In a heavy nonstick skillet, brown the ground turkey over medium-high heat, stirring often, until well browned and crumbly. Discard any fat. Add the tomatoes, onion, celery, jalapeño, garlic, curry powder, ginger, thyme, salt (if using), and pepper. Cook, stirring, until most of the liquid evaporates.

Mix together the cornstarch, sherry, and broth. Add to the skillet and cook, stirring, until the mixture boils and thickens, about 3 minutes. Remove from the stove to cool slightly.

Open the biscuit can and place the biscuits on a lightly floured work surface. Roll each biscuit into a 5-inch circle.

Spoon about ¼ cup of the cooled turkey mixture onto the center of each round. Flatten slightly with the back of a spoon. Lightly brush the outside edge of the dough with water. Fold half of the biscuit dough over the filling to make a half-circle. Press the edges together to seal, then crimp the edge with a fork.

Using a wide spatula, transfer the patties to an ungreased baking sheet, placing them 2 inches apart. Bake for 12 to 14 minutes, until puffed and nicely browned. Serve hot or warm.

Makes 5 patties.

PER 1-PATTY SERVING: 177 calories (33% calories from fat), 6 g total fat (1.7 g saturated fat), 13 g protein, 16 g carbohydrates, 1 g dietary fiber, 28 mg cholesterol, 354 mg sodium

JOSLIN EXCHANGES: 1½ very low fat protein, 1 carbohydrate (1 bread/starch)

French Sautéed Turkey Sandwich

Sandwiches are a favorite quick and easy supper at our houses, particularly when we've had a heavier lunch than usual. Here we've modified a recipe for *croque monsieur*, a French-style ham and cheese sandwich that is dipped in egg before being sautéed in butter.

Our lightened version uses leftover turkey breast or store-bought skinless, low-salt turkey breast. We also use thinly sliced whole wheat bread for fiber and texture—and, most of all, for its rich nutty taste.

4 ounces thinly sliced turkey breast
6 thin slices (4 ounces) fresh tomato
4 thin slices 100% whole wheat bread
½ teaspoon coarse-grain mustard
¼ cup egg substitute, diluted with 2 tablespoons water
butter-flavored cooking spray

Divide the turkey and tomatoes equally between 2 slices of bread. Spread the remaining 2 slices with mustard. Place on top of the filled bread.

Place the combined egg substitute and water in a shallow baking dish large enough to hold both sandwiches. Add the sandwiches and carefully turn them over once, until the egg mixture is absorbed.

Coat a large heavy-bottomed nonstick skillet with cooking spray. Cook the sandwiches over medium-high heat until the bottom is browned. Turn carefully and gently press down with a spatula. Continue cooking until the second side is browned.

Makes 2 servings.

PER SERVING: 214 calories (7% calories from fat), 2 g total fat (0.2 g saturated), 26 g protein, 24 g carbohydrates, 4 g dietary fiber, 47 mg cholesterol, 331 mg sodium

JOSLIN EXCHANGES: 3 very low fat protein, 1½ carbohydrate (1½ bread/starch)

Turkey Sloppy Joes

When you purchase ground turkey, read the label to be sure it doesn't contain any turkey skin. Most supermarkets sell ground white meat turkey with no by-products, but if the fat content is higher than 8 percent, buy a turkey or chicken breast. You can have your butcher remove and discard the skin and grind the turkey or chicken for you, wrapping it in 8-ounce packages for your freezer.

8 ounces extra-lean ground white meat turkey
¼ cup frozen chopped onion
1 tablespoon minced celery
1 medium green bell pepper, diced
1 6-ounce can low-sodium tomato sauce
1 teaspoon malt vinegar
1 teaspoon Worcestershire sauce
2 cloves garlic, minced, or ¼ teaspoon garlic powder
freshly ground pepper to taste
2 Kaiser rolls, split and toasted

Crumble the turkey in a large nonstick skillet. Cook over medium-high heat, stirring often, until the turkey is no longer pink, about 3 minutes. Drain any fat from the pan.

Lower the heat and stir in the remaining ingredients except the Kaiser rolls. Cover and simmer for 15 minutes.

Divide the turkey mixture between the Kaiser rolls. Serve immediately.

Makes 2 servings.

PER SERVING: 370 calories (10% calories from fat), 4 g total fat (0.4 g saturated fat), 36 g protein, 52 g carbohydrates, 3 g dietary fiber, 70 mg cholesterol, 635 mg sodium

JOSLIN EXCHANGES: 4 very low fat protein, 2½ carbohydrate (2½ bread/starch), 2 vegetable

Turkey Stroganoff

The original recipe for this late-1940s gourmet dish is rich with butter and sour cream. Modifying it for today's low-fat diet removes calories but keeps its deliciously succulent flavor. This dish benefits from being made ahead of time and reheating over low heat because the sauce improves with time.

8 ounces turkey tenderloin, cut on the diagonal against the grain into thin slices,
    white membrane discarded
1 teaspoon all-purpose flour
butter-flavored cooking spray
¼ cup frozen chopped onion
1 cup sliced button mushrooms
½ cup low-sodium canned chicken broth
⅓ cup fat-free sour cream
½ teaspoon Worcestershire sauce
1 teaspoon tomato paste
1 teaspoon fresh lemon juice

Toss the turkey with the flour. Lightly coat a large nonstick skillet with cooking spray. Add the turkey, a few pieces at a time (do not crowd the pan). Cook over high heat, turning once, until lightly browned on both sides, about 2 minutes. Transfer the turkey pieces to a plate and keep warm.

Turn heat to low. Place the onion and mushrooms in the same skillet and cook, stirring, until the onions have wilted, about 4 minutes. Stir in the broth, sour cream, Worcestershire sauce, tomato paste, and lemon juice. Continue to cook and stir until the sour cream has blended into the sauce. Do not allow the mixture to boil once the sour cream has been added, or the sauce may separate. Return the browned turkey to the skillet and simmer, uncovered, until heated through, about 3 minutes.

Makes 2 servings.

PER SERVING: 181 calories (10% calories from fat), 2 g total fat (0.6 g saturated fat), 31 g protein, 11 g carbohydrates, 1 g dietary fiber, 70 mg cholesterol, 152 mg sodium

JOSLIN EXCHANGES: 4 very low fat protein, 1 carbohydrate (1 bread/starch)

Grilled Cornish Game Hens, Thai Style

We do a lot of grilling—between us we have two indoor grills and five outside grills (gas and charcoal) for various uses. It is the simplest and fastest way to prepare a tasty meal. ⸎ Rock Cornish game hens are particularly well suited for this method of cooking. A game hen usually weighs about 1 pound and comes two hens to a package. Since half of a hen is an ample serving per person, ask your butcher to split the hens lengthwise and freezer-wrap the extra hen for another meal. Be sure not to eat the skin, or you'll be adding 56 calories and 6 grams of fat to each serving. ⸎ While the hens are grilling, make a couple of Grilled Vegetable Skewers (page 191). Then all you'll need to finish the meal is a mixed green salad.

1 1-pound Cornish game hen, split in half lengthwise
1 clove garlic, minced
½ teaspoon ground ginger
freshly ground pepper to taste

Thai relish:

2 tablespoons minced red onion
2 tablespoons minced cilantro
2 tablespoons minced fresh mint
1 red or green fresh jalapeño chile pepper, seeded and minced
2 teaspoons light brown sugar
2 teaspoons grated lemon zest
2 cloves garlic, minced
½ tablespoon minced fresh ginger
1½ tablespoons reduced-sodium soy sauce
2 tablespoons fresh lemon juice

Start a charcoal or gas grill, or preheat the broiler.

Rinse the game hen and remove all visible fat. Pat dry with paper towels. In a small bowl, combine the garlic, ginger, and pepper. Rub this mixture evenly over the hen halves.

Grill or broil, 4 to 6 inches from the medium-hot heat source. Turn the hen halves every 5 minutes for even browning, allowing 25 to 30 minutes total cooking time. The hen is done when the meat near the thighbone is no longer pink; cut to test.

Meanwhile, in the bowl of a food processor, combine the Thai relish ingredients. Pulse until finely minced. Spoon into a small bowl.

To serve, arrange the hen halves on 2 serving plates. Pass the relish to spoon over them. Serve at once.

Makes 2 servings.

PER SERVING: 264 calories (32% calories from fat), 9 g total fat (2.1 g saturated fat), 32 g protein, 9 g carbohydrates, 1 g dietary fiber, 100 mg cholesterol, 469 mg sodium

JOSLIN EXCHANGES: 4½ very low fat meat, ½ carbohydrate (½ bread/starch)

Grilled Cornish Hens, Provence-Style

If your taste is for less spicy food, rub the split hen with a mixture of ½ teaspoon of Dijon-style mustard, ½ teaspoon of minced garlic, ½ tablespoon of red wine vinegar, and ¼ teaspoon of olive oil. Grill as directed above. Serve with your favorite purchased steak sauce (but go easy on the steak sauce if you're on a sodium-restricted diet).

PER SERVING: 229 calories (39% calories from fat), 10 g total fat (2.2 g saturated fat), 31 g protein, 1 g carbohydrate, 0 dietary fiber, 100 mg cholesterol, 118 mg sodium

JOSLIN EXCHANGES: 4½ very low fat protein

Warm Duck and Lentil Salad with Mango Dressing

If you prefer, substitute boneless, skinless chicken breasts for the duck in this elegant meal. Mangoes are easy to dice if you peel one side at a time and make cuts perpendicular to the large flat seed and then slice across the cuts. Remember to select a mango that is ripe. Look for one that is soft to the touch and has yellow and red coloring on the green skin.

*12 ounces boneless duck breast, 8 ounces with the skin and fat removed, scored with a
    sharp knife in a diamond pattern*
3 tablespoons reduced-sodium teriyaki sauce

Lentil salad:

½ cup red lentils
2 cups water
½ cup frozen chopped onion
1 bay leaf
½ teaspoon crushed dried thyme
2 cloves garlic, minced, or ¼ teaspoon garlic powder
¼ teaspoon salt (optional)
freshly ground pepper to taste

Mango dressing:

1 8-ounce ripe mango, peeled and diced
1 tablespoon balsamic vinegar
1 tablespoon olive oil
1 tablespoon water
freshly ground pepper to taste
1 tablespoon chopped fresh mint or 1 teaspoon crushed dried

5 ounces mesclun, mixed young baby greens, or your favorite lettuces, torn into bite-
*   sized pieces*
extra mint leaves for garnish (optional)

Remove the skin and all visible fat from the duck breast and place in a nonreactive dish with the teriyaki sauce.

Wash the lentils and place with the water, in a pot that has a cover. Add the onion, bay leaf, thyme, garlic, salt (if using), and pepper. Bring to a simmer, cover, and cook for 15 minutes. Do not overcook or the lentils will become mushy. Drain the lentils and return to the pot, discarding the bay leaf. Set aside.

While the lentils are cooking, make the dressing. Peel and dice the mango and place in a small bowl. Add the vinegar, oil, water, pepper, and mint. Stir to combine well.

Light a charcoal or gas grill, or preheat the broiler.

When the lentils are almost done, remove the duck from the teriyaki sauce. Discard the sauce. Grill or broil, 4 to 6 inches from the heat source, for 2 to 3 minutes per side, turning once. Do not overcook; the duck meat should be rosy pink inside. If you prefer your duck more well done, increase the grilling time, but no more than an additional minute per side or the duck may become tough. Transfer the duck to a carving board. Let stand while you make the salad.

Place half of the mesclun on each of 2 serving plates. Top with a rounded mound of the lentils. Thinly slice the duck breast and arrange on top of the lentils, fanning out the slices. Stir the mango dressing and spoon around the duck. Decorate with extra mint leaves if desired and serve.

Makes 2 servings.

PER SERVING: 535 calories (25% calories from fat), 15 g total fat (2.6 g saturated fat), 40 g protein, 60 g carbohydrates, 12 g dietary fiber, 88 mg cholesterol, 746 mg sodium

JOSLIN EXCHANGES: 4 low fat protein, 3½ carbohydrate (2½ bread/starch, 1 fruit), 1 vegetable, 1 fat

{ Lean Meats }

Grilled Marinated Flank Steak, Chinese Style

Fresh ginger is frequently used when making Asian food. A tropical or subtropical plant grown for its gnarled root, fresh ginger must be peeled before using. Some cooks suggest freezing fresh ginger; however, it becomes mushy when defrosted and must be added to the dish in a frozen state. ❡ We suggest you buy a small piece and store any extra unpeeled ginger, tightly wrapped in plastic wrap, in the refrigerator for up to one week. You can also store any remaining peeled ginger in a screw-top glass jar, covered with dry sherry; refrigerate for up to three weeks. Once you begin to cook with this pungent spice, you won't have to worry about long-term storage.

Marinade:

3 tablespoons dry sherry or Chinese cooking wine
2 tablespoons fresh orange juice
2 tablespoons reduced-sodium soy sauce
2 cloves garlic, minced, or ¼ teaspoon garlic powder
2 scallions (white part only), finely chopped
1½-inch piece fresh ginger, minced
1 teaspoon grated orange zest
⅛ teaspoon crushed red pepper flakes (optional)

8 ounces flank steak

In a 1-cup measuring cup, combine the dry sherry, orange juice, soy sauce, garlic, scallions, ginger, orange zest, and red pepper flakes (if using).

Using a sharp knife, lightly score the flank steak with diagonal lines about ⅛ inch deep. Place in a shallow glass baking dish and pour on the marinade. Turn once to coat evenly. Let stand at room temperature for 15 minutes.

Light a charcoal or gas grill, or preheat the broiler.

Remove the steak from the marinade and grill or broil 4 to 5 inches from the heat source, turning frequently. Baste with the marinade until cooked to desired doneness, about 5 to 7 minutes for medium-rare.

Transfer the meat to a carving board and allow to rest for a few minutes before slicing on the diagonal into very thin slices.

Makes 2 servings.

PER SERVING: 284 calories (37% calories from fat), 12 g total fat (5.0 g saturated fat), 33 g protein, 7 g carbohydrates, <1 g dietary fiber, 76 mg cholesterol, 604 mg sodium

JOSLIN EXCHANGES: 4½ low fat protein, ½ carbohydrate (½ bread/starch)

Quick-Cooking Swiss Steak

Changing the cut of beef from round steak to cube steak makes for quick cooking, allowing us to enjoy this homey dish more often. Serve the steak over cooked yolk-free wide egg noodles that have been tossed with ¼ teaspoon of poppy seeds.

olive oil cooking spray
½ cup frozen chopped onion
2 cloves garlic, minced, or ¼ teaspoon garlic powder
1 medium green bell pepper, roughly chopped
2 5-ounce pieces cubed beef round steak
½ teaspoon Worcestershire sauce
1 tablespoon all-purpose flour
freshly ground pepper to taste
1 14½-ounce can no-salt-added whole tomatoes, drained
1 tablespoon chopped fresh basil or ½ teaspoon crushed dried
1 tablespoon fresh thyme leaves or ½ teaspoon crushed dried
¼ teaspoon ground cloves

Lightly coat a nonstick skillet with cooking spray. Add the onion, garlic, and bell pepper, and sauté over medium-high heat until the onion is just wilted, about 2 minutes. Transfer the vegetables to a plate.

Rub the Worcestershire sauce into the cube steaks and dust with flour. Season with pepper. In the same skillet, brown the steaks over medium-high heat for 1 minute per side. Turn the heat to low and return the onion-pepper mixture to the pan. Add the drained tomatoes, breaking them up with a wooden spoon. Sprinkle with the herbs and cloves. Bring to a simmer, cover, and cook for 10 minutes.

Transfer the meat to a heated serving platter and keep warm. Turn the heat to high and reduce the sauce for 3 minutes, stirring frequently. Pour the sauce and vegetables over the steaks and serve.

Makes 2 servings.

PER SERVING: 321 calories (26% calories from fat), 9 g total fat (3.4 g saturated fat), 37 g protein, 23 g carbohydrates, 6 g dietary fiber, 94 mg cholesterol, 126 mg sodium

JOSLIN EXCHANGES: 4 low fat protein, ½ carbohydrate (½ bread/starch), 3 vegetable

Tenderloin Tips and Mushrooms over Mashed Potatoes

Tenderloin tips come from the tail of the tenderloin of beef. Because it is not used for Châteaubriand, tournedos, or filet mignon, tenderloin tips are often half the price but have the same flavor and texture of the pricier cuts.

8 ounces tenderloin tail, cut into thin slices about 2 inches in length
6 ounces fresh button mushroom caps, quartered
1 scallion (white part only), thinly sliced
½ cup low-sodium canned beef broth
2 tablespoons white wine, dry sherry, or additional beef broth
1 teaspoon Dijon mustard
1 tablespoon fresh tarragon or 1 teaspoon crushed dried
1 tablespoon chopped fresh parsley
freshly ground pepper to taste

Mashed potatoes:

⅓ cup skim milk mixed with 1 cup water
1 cup instant mashed potatoes
1 tablespoon reduced-fat margarine
⅛ teaspoon garlic powder
freshly ground pepper to taste
chopped fresh chives or scallion tops for garnish (optional)

Place a large nonstick skillet over high heat for 30 seconds. Add the tenderloin tips and sear for 1 minute on each side for medium-rare, turning once. Add the mushrooms and scallion; cook, stirring, for 2 minutes. Transfer the meat and mushrooms to a plate and keep warm.

Stir into the same skillet the beef broth, wine, mustard, tarragon, parsley, and pepper. Bring to a boil and cook, stirring constantly and scraping up any browned bits, until the sauce reduces to a syrup consistency, about 3 to 4 minutes. Return the beef and mushrooms to the sauce. Keep warm while preparing the mashed potatoes.

In a medium saucepan, bring the milk-water mixture to a boil. Stir in the potatoes, margarine, garlic powder, and pepper. Whip by hand until smooth.

Make a ring of mashed potatoes on each dinner plate and fill with half of the tenderloin tips. Top with some of the sauce. Sprinkle with chopped chives if desired and serve.

Makes 2 servings.

PER SERVING: 393 calories (40% calories from fat), 17 g total fat (5.6 g saturated fat), 38 g protein, 21 g carbohydrates, 1 g dietary fiber, 98 mg cholesterol, 393 mg sodium

JOSLIN EXCHANGES: 3½ medium fat protein, 1 carbohydrate (1 bread/starch), 1 vegetable

Beef and Tomato Stir-Fry with Couscous

This delightful combination of flavors goes together in minutes. If you have fresh mint, use it. If not, pull some chopped parsley out of the freezer (see page 84) to use in the marinade.

> 6 ounces lean boneless top sirloin, cut 1 inch thick and all fat removed
> ¼ cup dry red wine or low-sodium canned beef broth
> 2 tablespoons orange juice
> 1 tablespoon red wine vinegar
> 1 tablespoon minced fresh mint or flat-leaf parsley
> 1 teaspoon minced fresh ginger or ⅛ teaspoon ground ginger
> 1 clove garlic, minced, or ⅛ teaspoon garlic powder
> 1 cup fat-free reduced-sodium canned chicken broth
> ⅔ cup instant couscous
> ¼ teaspoon ground cumin
> 1 teaspoon canola oil
> 1 medium onion, cut in half and then thinly sliced
> 8 large (about 4 ounces) red or yellow cherry tomatoes
> mint sprigs for garnish (optional)

Slice the beef across the grain into slices about ⅛ inch wide and 2 inches long. Place in a medium bowl. In a glass measuring cup, mix together the red wine, orange juice, vinegar, mint, ginger, and garlic. Pour over the steak and stir to coat evenly. Cover and refrigerate for 15 minutes.

Place the broth in a small saucepan that has a cover. Bring to a boil over high heat. Stir in the couscous and cumin, cover, and remove from the heat. Let stand until the liquid has been absorbed, about 5 minutes. Keep warm, fluffing occasionally with a fork.

Heat the oil in a wok or large nonstick skillet over high heat. Add the onion and stir-fry until it is soft, about 2 minutes. Add the tomatoes and stir-fry for 3 minutes. Transfer the onion-tomato mixture to a plate.

Using a slotted spoon, transfer the beef strips to the wok. Reserve the marinade. Stir-fry the beef until cooked to desired doneness (cut to test), about 2 to 3 minutes for medium-rare. Return the onion-tomato mixture to the wok and add the reserved marinade. Continue to cook, stirring gently, until the mixture boils.

To serve, mound the couscous in the center of a serving platter. Spoon the beef and tomato mixture around the couscous and garnish with mint sprigs if desired.

Makes 2 servings.

PER SERVING: 479 calories (22% calories from fat), 11 g total fat (2.9 g saturated fat), 33 g protein, 60 g carbohydrates, 4 g dietary fiber, 66 mg cholesterol, 118 mg sodium

JOSLIN EXCHANGES: 3 low fat protein, 3 carbohydrate (3 bread/starch), 3 vegetable

Stuffed Burgers

Here we have a delicious twist to the hamburger: a filling that oozes from the inside out. These are so good that the bun and other trimmings are optional. (If you elect to serve these on a bun with tomato, lettuce, and so forth, check the Joslin Exchanges, page 249, for the added exchanges.)

8 ounces extra-lean ground sirloin
1 tablespoon minced red onion
1 teaspoon minced fresh basil
½ teaspoon Dijon mustard
dash chili powder
½ ounce part-skim mozzarella or reduced-fat sharp cheddar cheese, cut into 2 chunks

Light a charcoal or gas grill, or preheat the broiler.

In a small bowl, gently mix all the ingredients except the mozzarella cheese. Divide the mixture in half. Form each half around a piece of the cheese, and shape into thick patties.

Grill or broil the hamburgers, 4 inches from the heat source, to desired doneness, about 7 minutes per side for medium-rare, turning once.

Makes 2 servings.

PER SERVING: 195 calories (39% calories from fat), 8 g total fat (3.4 g saturated fat), 28 g protein, 1 g carbohydrates, <1 g dietary fiber, 80 cholesterol, 126 mg sodium

JOSLIN EXCHANGES: 4 very low fat protein

Variations: Other Stuffings for Burgers

In place of the mozzarella cheese, use one of these stuffings. We've calculated your added exchanges and calories.

- A tablespoon of sautéed minced onion seasoned with crushed dried thyme. Same exchanges, 18 fewer calories.

- A few slices of sautéed mushrooms seasoned with crushed dried sage. Same exchanges, 18 fewer calories.

- A thin slice of plum tomato. Same exchanges, 18 fewer calories.

- A chunk of pineapple, fresh or canned in its own juice. Same exchanges, 18 fewer calories.

- A piece of rehydrated sun-dried tomato. Same exchanges, 23 fewer calories.

- A spoonful of cooked lentils. Adds ½ carbohydrate (½ bread/starch) exchange and 9 calories.

- A tablespoon of Lower-Fat Goat Cheese (page 33). Same exchanges, same calories.

- Cooked sliced potatoes. Adds ½ carbohydrate (½ bread/starch) exchange and 11 calories.

Mexicali Stuffed Peppers

Using the microwave makes this meal possible to prepare in minutes. Corn replaces the usual rice for an interesting change in flavor and texture, but feel free to use left-over rice or canned beans in place of the corn as long as you note how this will affect the exchange values (see Joslin Exchanges, page 249).

6 ounces extra-lean ground sirloin
½ cup frozen chopped onion
1 clove garlic, minced, or ⅛ teaspoon garlic powder
½ teaspoon Worcestershire sauce
1 8-ounce can reduced-sodium tomato sauce
1 cup frozen corn kernels
2 tablespoons minced fresh cilantro or flat-leaf parsley
1 tablespoon golden raisins
1 canned jalapeño chile, finely minced (optional)
freshly ground pepper to taste
2 medium green bell peppers (about 6 ounces each)
2 tablespoons shredded reduced-fat Monterey Jack cheese

Crumble the beef into a large nonstick skillet and cook over medium-high heat until the meat is browned, about 5 minutes. Drain off any fat. Return the beef to the stove and add the onion, garlic, and Worcestershire sauce. Cook, stirring, for 1 minute. Stir in 2 tablespoons of the tomato sauce, corn, cilantro, raisins, jalapeño (if using), and pepper. Bring to a slow simmer and cook, uncovered, while you prepare the peppers for stuffing.

With a sharp knife, cut and discard the stem ends of the peppers. Cut in half lengthwise and remove the membranes and seeds. Place the peppers, cut side down, in a microwave-safe baking dish. Cover with waxed paper and cook on HIGH for 3 minutes. Remove from the microwave and drain the peppers.

Stuff the peppers with the beef mixture and arrange in the baking dish, stuffing side up. Pour the remaining tomato sauce on the stuffed peppers, cover with waxed paper, and cook for 4 minutes on HIGH. Turn the dish and sprinkle with the cheese. Cook, uncovered, for another 3 minutes on HIGH. Remove the dish from the microwave and let stand for 2 minutes before serving.

Makes 2 servings.

PER SERVING: 371 calories (19% calories from fat), 9 g total fat (3.6 g saturated fat), 35 g protein, 45 g carbohydrates, 8 g dietary fiber, 81 mg cholesterol, 174 mg sodium

JOSLIN EXCHANGES: 3½ very low fat protein, 2 carbohydrate (2 bread/starch), 3 vegetable

Spud-Stuffed Mini Beef Loaves

If you haven't discovered tomato paste in a tube, you'll find it alongside the canned variety at your supermarket. It's richly flavored and perfect for recipes like this where you need only a teaspoon or so. Store the tube in the refrigerator; it'll stay fresh for months. ❡ This recipe proves that your microwave is good for more than boiling water and defrosting frozen foods. It allows you to make short work of this comfort food.

6 ounces extra-lean ground sirloin
1 clove garlic, minced, or ⅛ teaspoon garlic powder
½ teaspoon onion powder
2 teaspoons tomato paste plus ¼ teaspoon (optional)
1 teaspoon Dijon mustard
¼ teaspoon Worcestershire sauce plus ¼ teaspoon (optional)
¼ teaspoon crushed dried marjoram
¼ teaspoon crushed dried thyme
⅛ teaspoon crushed dried sage
¼ teaspoon kosher salt (optional)
freshly ground pepper to taste

2 tablespoons quick-cooking oatmeal (not instant)
¼ cup plus 1 tablespoon egg substitute
butter-flavored cooking spray
½ cup potato flakes (with no added fats or flavorings)
⅓ cup boiling water
1 tablespoon chopped fresh parsley for garnish (optional)

In a large bowl, combine the ground sirloin, garlic, onion powder, tomato paste, mustard, Worcestershire sauce, marjoram, thyme, sage, salt (if using), pepper, oatmeal, and ¼ cup egg substitute. Mix until just combined. Do not overmix or the mixture will become too dense. Form the mixture into 2 loaves of equal size.

Lightly coat a microwave-safe baking dish with cooking spray. Place the loaves in the baking dish.

In a small bowl, mix the potato flakes with the water. (The potatoes will be stiffer than usual.) Add the remaining 1 tablespoon of egg substitute and pepper to taste.

With your finger, make a trench down the middle on the top of each meat loaf, leaving an equal amount of the beef all around. Stuff the trench with the potato mixture. Pull and mold the beef up and over the potatoes, trying to enclose them completely. Lightly coat with cooking spray. If you wish, combine the optional Worcestershire sauce and tomato paste, and spoon a little on top of each loaf.

Cover the baking dish with waxed paper and cook in the microwave for 5 minutes on MEDIUM HIGH. Remove the baking dish and rearrange the meat loaves in the dish to make sure all sides are exposed to the outside of the dish. (The easiest way to do this is to switch places and turn.) Cover once again with waxed paper and cook another 5 minutes on MEDIUM HIGH. Remove the dish from the oven, allow to sit for 3 minutes, then garnish with fresh parsley if desired before serving.

Makes 2 servings.

PER SERVING: 262 calories (26% calories from fat), 8 g total fat grams (2.8 g saturated fat), 32 g protein, 16 g carbohydrates, 2 g dietary fiber, 76 mg cholesterol, 244 mg sodium

JOSLIN EXCHANGE: 4 very low fat protein, 1 carbohydrate (1 bread/starch)

Pork Burritos with Papaya Salsa

These burritos are missing the customary cheese, refried beans, and guacamole, but you certainly won't find them lacking in flavor or taste appeal. Today's well-trimmed pork tenderloin competes with chicken as a lean, low-cholesterol meat, making it perfect for these low-fat burritos. The salsa is made with papaya; you can also use half of a ripe mango or a medium-firm, ripe peach or nectarine.

1 tablespoon fresh lemon juice
1 tablespoon fresh lime juice
1 tablespoon fresh orange juice
5 sprigs fresh cilantro
½ jalapeño chile pepper, seeded and minced
dash cayenne pepper
⅓ pound pork tenderloin, trimmed of all fat

Papaya salsa:

½ firm, ripe papaya (about 6 ounces)
½ jalapeño chile pepper, seeded and minced
1 tablespoon minced cilantro
1 scallion (white part only), thinly sliced
1 tablespoon fresh lime juice
1 tablespoon white wine vinegar
2 drops hot pepper sauce

vegetable oil cooking spray
2 10-inch 98% fat-free flour tortillas
2 large romaine lettuce leaves, cut into strips
2 tablespoons fat-free sour cream

In a medium bowl, combine the juices, cilantro, jalapeño, and cayenne. Cut the pork tenderloin on the diagonal into ¼-inch slices, then cut each slice into several thin strips. Add to the juice mixture and toss to coat evenly. Cover and let stand for 15 minutes.

Meanwhile, scoop out and discard the seeds of the papaya. Peel and cut into ¼-inch cubes. In a small bowl, combine the papaya with the remaining salsa ingredients. Set aside until ready to use.

Lightly coat a large nonstick skillet or wok with cooking spray. Add the pork mixture and stir-fry over medium-high heat until the pork is lightly browned on the outside and no longer pink in the center (cut to test), about 8 minutes.

Using tongs, toast the tortillas directly over the burner at medium heat for about 30 seconds, turning once.

On the bottom third of each tortilla, place several strips of pork, several strips of lettuce, and 2 tablespoons of the salsa. Roll up and serve with the remaining salsa and sour cream.

Makes 2 servings.

PER SERVING: 298 calories (11% calories from fat), 4 g total fat grams (1 g saturated fat), 22 g protein, 48 g carbohydrates, 9 g dietary fiber, 45 mg cholesterol, 370 mg sodium

JOSLIN EXCHANGES: 2 very low fat protein, 3 carbohydrate (2 bread/starch, 1 fruit)

Roasted Pork Tenderloin with Mustard Herb Rub

Start this recipe the night before and let the tenderloin marinate overnight. The next day it oven-roasts in about 30 minutes, giving you just enough time to prepare the rest of the meal. Pork tenderloins come two to a package. Wrap and freeze one for later in the month. From the one you roast you'll still have enough leftovers to make a sandwich the next day.

1 tablespoon balsamic vinegar
1 tablespoon Dijon mustard
¼ teaspoon crushed dried oregano
¼ teaspoon crushed dried rosemary
¼ teaspoon crushed dried sage
1 10-ounce pork tenderloin

In a small bowl, combine the vinegar, mustard, oregano, rosemary, and sage. Spread over the pork tenderloin, coating all sides. Place in a self-sealing plastic bag and refrigerate overnight or for at least 8 hours.

Preheat the oven to 375°F. Bake the tenderloin on a rack in a roasting pan for 20 to 25 minutes, until an instant-reading meat thermometer registers 160°F. When the pork is done, remove from the oven and let stand for 5 minutes. Thinly slice on the diagonal. Arrange 3 slices on each of 2 dinner plates.

Makes 3 servings.

PER SERVING: 138 calories (28% calories from fat), 4 g total fat grams (1.3 g saturated fat), 22 g protein, 2 g carbohydrates, 0 dietary fiber, 60 mg cholesterol, 170 mg sodium

JOSLIN EXCHANGES: 3 very low fat protein

Jerked Pork Skewers with Orange Sauce

Jerk is an aromatic seasoning that is well known throughout the Caribbean. Although there are some very good jerk seasonings available at specialty food stores, it is easily made from scratch for pennies. ¶ Serve this with Couscous with Currants and Walnuts (page 187). The orange sauce complements both.

8 ounces pork tenderloin, trimmed of all fat

Jerk Marinade:

¼ teaspoon ground allspice
¼ teaspoon ground cinnamon
⅛ teaspoon ground cloves
⅛ teaspoon ground ginger
⅛ teaspoon ground nutmeg
1 clove garlic, minced
1 teaspoon minced jalapeño chile pepper
1 tablespoon fresh orange juice

Orange sauce:

2 tablespoons plain nonfat yogurt
3 tablespoons fresh orange juice
1 teaspoon minced orange zest
1 tablespoon finely minced fresh cilantro or flat-leaf parsley
dash cayenne pepper

Light a charcoal or gas grill, or preheat the broiler.

Cut the pork into 1-inch cubes. In a medium bowl, combine the ingredients for the jerk marinade. Add the pork and stir to coat evenly. Cover with plastic wrap and refrigerate for 15 minutes.

Meanwhile, combine the ingredients for the orange sauce and whisk until smooth. Set aside.

Thread the pork on skewers. Place on a lightly greased grill or broiler, 4 to 6 inches from the heat source. Cook, turning often, until the pork is well browned and no longer pink in the center, 7 to 10 minutes. Cut to test. Serve the pork with the orange sauce.

Makes 2 servings.

PER SERVING: 188 calories (28% calories from fat), 6 g total fat grams (2 g saturated fat), 27 g protein, 6 g carbohydrates, 0 dietary fiber, 80 mg cholesterol, 89 mg sodium

JOSLIN EXCHANGES: 4 very low fat protein, ½ carbohydrate (½ fruit)

Pork Chops with Apricots and Prunes

In this recipe the play of savory and sweet flavors elevates lowly boneless pork chops to the sublime. Coarsely ground pepper and balsamic vinegar are added to the sauce at the end, further adding a bit of heat and spice. Best of all, the dish takes only 25 minutes from start to finish.

4 dried apricots, cut into thin strips
4 dried pitted prunes, cut into thin strips
2 tablespoons minced red onion
¼ teaspoon minced garlic
2 tablespoons good-quality whiskey, such as Jack Daniel's
2 4-ounce boneless center-cut pork chops, cut ¾ inch thick and trimmed of all fat
salt (optional)
freshly ground pepper to taste
olive oil cooking spray
1 cup fat-free reduced-sodium canned chicken broth
½ teaspoon grated lemon zest
¼ teaspoon coarsely ground pepper, or to taste
1 teaspoon balsamic vinegar

In a small bowl, combine the apricots, prunes, onion, garlic, and whiskey. Stir to mix well. Set aside.

Season the pork with salt (if using) and pepper. Lightly coat a nonstick sauté pan with cooking spray. Place over medium heat. Add the pork and sauté for 3 to 4 minutes per side, until lightly browned and cooked. Transfer to a plate, cover with foil, and keep warm.

Add the fruit-whiskey mixture to the same pan. Cook, stirring constantly, until the mixture boils, scraping up any browned bits on the bottom of the pan. Add the broth and lemon zest. Continue to cook, stirring occasionally, until the sauce is slightly thickened, about 8 minutes. Stir in the coarsely ground pepper and vinegar. Return the pork to the pan and continue to cook for another minute or so, until the pork is well coated with sauce.

To serve, place the chops on dinner plates and spoon the sauce around them.

Makes 2 servings.

PER SERVING: 296 calories (22% calories from fat), 7 g total fat grams (2.6 g saturated fat), 28 g protein, 22 g carbohydrates, 2 g dietary fiber, 73 mg cholesterol, 336 mg sodium

JOSLIN EXCHANGES: 4 very low fat protein, 1½ carbohydrate (1½ fruit)

Baby Lamb Chops with Mint Vinaigrette

Years ago lamb chops were usually served with mint jelly. This updated version is light and much more flavorful. The vinaigrette mingles with the lamb juices on the plate to make a succulent sauce.

4 4-ounce rib lamb chops, cut about ¾ inch thick
¼ teaspoon chili powder
¼ teaspoon ground turmeric
⅛ teaspoon ground cinnamon
⅛ teaspoon salt (optional)
dash cayenne pepper
1 clove garlic, minced
1 teaspoon Dijon mustard

Mint vinaigrette:

1 tablespoon chopped fresh mint
½ teaspoon Dijon mustard
¼ teaspoon freshly ground pepper
1 tablespoon balsamic vinegar
1 teaspoon olive oil

Start a charcoal or gas grill, or preheat the broiler.

Trim off all fat from the lamb chops, leaving the bone in. In a small bowl, make a paste by combining the chili powder, turmeric, cinnamon, salt (if using), cayenne pepper, garlic, and mustard.

Grill or broil the lamb chops 4 inches from the heat source for 3 minutes. Turn and brush with the mustard mixture. Continue grilling for another 3½ to 4 minutes for medium-rare, or to desired doneness.

While the chops are grilling, combine the mint, mustard, pepper, and vinegar. Whisk in the olive oil.

To serve, place 2 chops on each of 2 dinner plates. Drizzle with the vinaigrette and serve at once.

Makes 2 servings.

PER SERVING: 240 calories (53% calories from fat), 14 g total fat grams (6.4 g saturated fat), 24 g protein, 4 g carbohydrates, 0 dietary fiber, 79 mg cholesterol, 172 mg sodium

JOSLIN EXCHANGES: 3½ medium fat protein

Lemon Veal with Mushrooms and Capers

We've added mushrooms to a piquant lemon-caper sauce for a quick, light version of the classic veal piccata. Serve this with Garlic Mashed Potatoes (page 181) and steamed asparagus for a meal worthy of company (after doubling or tripling the recipe). ❡ Most supermarkets sell mushrooms already cleaned and sliced, which saves kitchen time.

8 ounces veal scaloppine, cut into strips ¼ inch by 2 inches
1 shallot, minced, or 1 tablespoon minced red onion
¼ teaspoon paprika
⅛ teaspoon salt (optional)
freshly ground pepper to taste
1 teaspoon reduced-fat margarine
1 teaspoon olive oil
1 8-ounce package cleaned and sliced mushrooms
⅓ cup dry white wine or low-sodium canned chicken broth
1½ tablespoons fresh lemon juice
¼ teaspoon grated lemon zest
1 teaspoon capers, well drained

In a medium bowl, toss the veal with the shallot, paprika, salt (if using), and pepper.

Heat the margarine and oil in a large nonstick skillet over medium-high heat. Add the veal and cook, stirring, until the meat is no longer pink on the outside, about 2 to 3 minutes. Using a slotted spoon, transfer the meat to a plate.

Add the mushrooms to the same skillet and cook, stirring, until they are soft and the pan liquid is almost gone. Scrape up any browned bits in the bottom of the skillet. Stir in the wine, lemon juice, lemon zest, and capers. Bring the mixture to a boil, stirring constantly. Return the veal to the skillet and cook for another minute, turning the veal to coat all sides.

To serve, divide the veal between 2 dinner plates. Top each serving with some of the sauce and serve at once.

Makes 2 servings.

PER SERVING: 228 calories (31% calories from fat), 8 g total fat grams (2.2 g saturated fat), 26 g protein, 8 g carbohydrates, 2 g dietary fiber, 88 mg cholesterol, 140 mg sodium

JOSLIN EXCHANGES: 3½ very low fat protein, 1 vegetable, 1 fat

{ One-Pot Meals }

Casseroles, Stews, Soups, Stir-Fries, Sandwiches, and Skillet Suppers

Scallops with Rotini and Pesto

This delicious dish is very pretty and goes together in a jiffy. If you can't find rotini, use any corkscrew pasta.

4 ounces rotini or other corkscrew pasta

Basil pesto

1 tablespoon chopped walnuts
2 cloves garlic, peeled
1 cup loosely packed fresh basil leaves
2 tablespoons fat-free reduced-sodium canned chicken broth
1 tablespoon fresh lemon juice

8 ounces bay scallops, rinsed and well drained
¼ teaspoon paprika
¼ teaspoon crushed dried basil
¼ teaspoon crushed dried thyme
1 clove garlic, minced
1 teaspoon canola oil
6 frozen artichoke hearts, thawed and cut in half
½ fresh lemon
salt (optional)
freshly ground pepper to taste

Bring 4 cups of water to a boil in a large pot over medium-high heat. Add the rotini and cook until al dente, 8 to 10 minutes, or cook according to package directions.

   To make the basil pesto: Place the walnuts, garlic, and basil in the bowl of a food processor. Turn on the machine and add 1 tablespoon of the chicken broth through the feed tube, then drizzle in the lemon juice to form a paste. Transfer the mixture to a small mixing bowl and whisk in the remaining tablespoon of chicken broth. Set aside.

In another small bowl, combine the scallops, paprika, dried basil, thyme, and garlic. Toss to coat the scallops evenly.

Heat the oil in a large nonstick skillet over medium-high heat. Add the scallop mixture and artichokes. Stir-fry for 2 to 3 minutes, until the scallops are opaque in the center (cut to test) and the artichokes are tender. Squeeze the lemon over the scallops and artichokes, and turn the heat to low.

When the pasta is done, drain well, reserving ¼ cup of the pasta cooking liquid. Add the pasta to the skillet and stir in the reserved pesto, tossing to coat evenly. If needed, add some of the reserved cooking liquid until the pasta is the desired consistency. Season with salt (if using) and pepper. Divide the pasta between 2 bowls and serve immediately.

Makes 2 servings.

PER SERVING: 429 calories (17% calories from fat), 8 g total fat (0.5 g saturated fat), 31 g protein, 51 g carbohydrates, 6 g dietary fiber, 102 mg cholesterol, 238 mg sodium

JOSLIN EXCHANGES: 3 very low fat protein, 3 carbohydrate (3 bread/starch), 1 vegetable, 1 fat

New England Fish Chowder

This comforting chowder will offset the effects of a chilly day. Serve it with crusty bread, and fresh pears or apples with a little fat-free sharp cheddar cheese for dessert. Supper couldn't be easier.

1 cup frozen chopped onion
¼ cup shredded carrot
¼ cup thinly sliced celery
2¼ cups fat-free reduced-sodium canned chicken broth
2 no-salt-added canned tomatoes, coarsely chopped
1 small zucchini, diced
1 small red potato, unpeeled and diced
¼ teaspoon crushed dried thyme
salt (optional)
freshly ground pepper
5 ounces fillet of sole, flounder, or orange roughy, cut into ½-inch pieces
1 tablespoon finely minced flat-leaf parsley for garnish (optional)
1 scallion (white part only), thinly sliced, for garnish (optional)

In a large pot, combine the onion, carrot, celery, and ¼ cup of the chicken broth. Bring to a boil and cook over medium-high heat until the onion is limp, about 2 minutes. Add the remaining broth, tomatoes, zucchini, potato, and thyme. Lower the heat, cover, and simmer until the vegetables are cooked, about 15 minutes. Taste and add salt (if using) and pepper.

Add the fish, cover, and continue to simmer until the fish is tender, about 5 minutes. Ladle the chowder into 2 soup bowls and sprinkle with parsley and scallion if desired.

Makes 2 servings.

PER SERVING: 184 calories (6% calories from fat), 1 g total fat (0.3 g saturated fat), 20 g protein, 25 g carbohydrates, 5 g dietary fiber, 34 mg cholesterol, 730 mg sodium

JOSLIN EXCHANGES: 2 very low fat protein, 1 carbohydrate (1 bread/starch), 2 vegetable

Snapper Stew with New Potatoes and Tomatoes

Fish stews are traditional in many cultures. Here we've taken it just a little south of the border, to Mexico.

4 small new red potatoes, halved
¼ cup frozen chopped onion
1 tablespoon dried celery flakes
1 clove garlic, minced, or ⅛ teaspoon garlic powder
1 small fresh jalapeño chile pepper, seeded and minced
4 button mushrooms, sliced
1 14½-ounce can no-salt-added diced tomatoes, drained well
½ cup clam juice or low-sodium canned chicken broth
3 tablespoons dry white wine or 1 tablespoon lemon juice
¼ teaspoon ground cumin
8 ounces boneless red snapper fillets, cut into 1½-inch cubes
1 tablespoon chopped fresh cilantro, or to taste

Place the potatoes in a covered microwave-safe bowl with 1 tablespoon of water. Cook on HIGH for 4 minutes, stirring once. Set aside.

In a medium nonstick skillet, sauté the onion, celery flakes, garlic, jalapeño, and mushrooms over medium-high heat for 1 minute. Add the tomatoes, clam juice, wine, cumin, and cooked potatoes. Simmer, uncovered, for 5 minutes, stirring once. Add the fish and continue to simmer, uncovered, until the fish is opaque, about 2 to 3 minutes.

Spoon the stew into 2 shallow soup bowls and sprinkle with cilantro if desired.

Makes 2 servings.

PER SERVING: 284 calories (8% calories from fat), 2 g total fat (0.4 g saturated fat), 28 g protein, 34 g carbohydrates, 6 g dietary fiber, 42 mg cholesterol, 242 mg sodium

JOSLIN EXCHANGES: 3 very low fat protein, 1 carbohydrate (1 bread/starch), 3 vegetable

Easy Chicken Cacciatore with Summer Squash

Cacciatore is usually a slow-cooked chicken dish. Here we've cut the cooking time by using frozen chopped vegetables and bite-sized pieces of chicken as well as bits of fresh squash. With its great flavor and easy preparation, this is a dish you'll serve again and again. ❡ To complete the meal in a northern Italian mode, grill store-bought nonfat polenta as an accompaniment.

olive oil cooking spray
8 ounces boneless, skinless chicken breast, cut into 1½-inch pieces
1 teaspoon flour
¼ cup dry red wine or low-sodium canned beef broth
6 button mushrooms, thinly sliced
¼ cup frozen chopped onion
½ cup frozen chopped green pepper
1 clove garlic, minced, or ⅛ teaspoon garlic powder
2 small yellow summer squash, quartered lengthwise and cut into 1-inch pieces
1 teaspoon celery flakes
½ teaspoon crushed dried Italian seasoning
½ bay leaf
1 14½-ounce can no-salt-added diced tomatoes
freshly ground pepper to taste
chopped fresh basil for garnish (optional)

Toss the chicken with the flour. Lightly coat a large nonstick skillet with cooking spray and place over high heat. Add the chicken pieces. Cook, stirring, until browned on all sides, about 2 minutes. Transfer the chicken to a platter.

Lower the heat to medium. Pour the wine into the pan and stir to loosen any bits of chicken left in the pan. Add the remaining ingredients and cook for 1 minute. Return the chicken to the pan, cover, and simmer for 10 minutes.

Using a slotted spoon, transfer the chicken and as many of the vegetables as possible to a serving platter and keep warm.

To thicken the sauce, remove the bay leaf, raise the heat to high, and boil the sauce, stirring constantly, about 2 minutes. Spoon the sauce over the chicken and vegetables, and sprinkle with basil if desired. Serve immediately.

Makes 2 servings.

PER SERVING: 227 calories (9% calories from fat), 2 g total fat (0.6 g saturated fat), 37 g protein, 15 g carbohydrates, 5 g dietary fiber, 83 mg cholesterol, 110 mg sodium

JOSLIN EXCHANGES: 4 very low fat protein, 3 vegetable

Chicken Tamale Pie

This is a fresh and contemporary version of tamale pie, using boneless chicken breasts instead of ground beef and pork sausage. The casserole can be made ahead, covered tightly, and refrigerated, ready to bake the next day. If refrigerated, set out for 30 minutes to bring to room temperature before baking or add an extra 10 to 15 minutes to the baking time. ❡ Serve with a platter of raw vegetables and a tall pitcher of iced tea for a quick and easy meal.

olive oil cooking spray
6 ounces boneless, skinless chicken fillets, cut into 1-inch pieces
1 large tomato, diced
½ cup frozen chopped onion
½ cup frozen chopped green pepper
¼ cup frozen corn kernels
1 clove garlic, minced, or ⅛ teaspoon garlic powder
½ to 1 tablespoon chili powder to taste
¼ teaspoon ground cumin
dash cayenne pepper
½ cup (2 ounces) shredded reduced-fat sharp cheddar cheese

Cornmeal crust:

½ cup fat-free reduced-sodium canned chicken broth
½ cup yellow cornmeal
⅛ teaspoon ground cumin
dash cayenne pepper

Preheat the oven to 450°F. Lightly coat a 1-quart casserole or ramekin that is at least 2 inches deep with cooking spray.

Lightly coat a large nonstick skillet with cooking spray. Place over medium heat and add the chicken pieces. Sauté until browned on all sides, about 5 minutes. Add the tomato, onion, green pepper, corn, garlic, chili powder, cumin, and cayenne pepper. Lower the heat and simmer, stirring occasionally, for 5 minutes. Transfer the chicken mixture to the prepared casserole and top with cheese.

While the meat is cooking, bring the broth to a boil in a medium saucepan over medium-high heat. Stir in the cornmeal, cumin, and cayenne pepper. Lower the heat to medium and cook, stirring, until the mixture thickens, about 3 minutes. Immediately top the chicken-cheese mixture with the cornmeal mixture, smoothing with the back of a spoon and making sure the cornmeal is evenly distributed over the chicken mixture.

Bake, uncovered, for 20 to 25 minutes, until the cornmeal topping is golden brown and the filling is bubbling. Serve at once.

Makes 2 servings.

PER SERVING: 374 calories (19% calories from fat), 8 g total fat (4.3 g saturated fat), 35 g protein, 42 g carbohydrates, 6 g dietary fiber, 71 mg cholesterol, 342 mg sodium

JOSLIN EXCHANGES: 4 very low fat protein, 2 carbohydrate (2 bread/starch), 2 vegetable

Chicken Ragout

This dish reminds us very much of the very simple sort of chicken dishes our mothers made when we were children. We're sure you'll see a similarity, too.

olive oil cooking spray
1 8-ounce boneless, skinless chicken breast, cut into thin strips
1 small onion, halved and thinly sliced
1½ cups low-sodium canned chicken broth
2 small red potatoes, scrubbed and quartered
2 medium plum tomatoes, quartered
½ cup frozen baby peas
¼ teaspoon dill weed
freshly ground pepper to taste
1 tablespoon grated Parmesan cheese

Lightly coat a large nonstick skillet with cooking spray. Add the chicken strips and onion. Sauté over medium-high heat for 5 minutes.

Stir in the chicken broth and add the potatoes. Lower the heat to medium, cover, and cook for 15 minutes, until the potatoes are just tender. Add the tomatoes and peas, and continue to cook, uncovered, for 5 minutes. Stir in the dill and season with pepper.

To serve, divide equally between 2 shallow soup plates and sprinkle with cheese.

Makes 2 servings.

PER SERVING: 276 calories (13% calories from fat), 4 g total fat (1.8 g saturated fat), 34 g protein, 26 g carbohydrate, 5 g dietary fiber, 72 mg cholesterol, 266 mg sodium

JOSLIN EXCHANGES: 4 very low fat protein, 1½ carbohydrate (1½ bread/starch), 1 vegetable

Chicken Gumbo

Throughout the South, many stewlike dishes that contain tomatoes and sweet peppers are called gumbos, but unless they contain okra, they're not the gumbo that is typical in New Orleans. ❡ This recipe has okra, but the dish is mild and light (it doesn't have any dark roux thickening), and not overly spicy-hot. Extra heat can always be added by passing the bottle of hot pepper sauce at the table. ❡ If you are having rice earlier in the week, make extra so that all you have to do is reheat it in the microwave.

olive oil cooking spray
4 ounces okra, stems removed, or 1 cup sliced thawed frozen okra
½ cup frozen chopped onion
¼ cup chopped red bell pepper
¼ cup chopped green bell pepper
1 clove garlic, minced
1¼ cups fat-free reduced-sodium canned chicken broth
1 14½-ounce can no-salt-added diced tomatoes
1 teaspoon fresh thyme leaves or ¼ teaspoon crushed dried
¼ teaspoon ground cumin
1 small bay leaf
2 5-ounce bone-in chicken thighs, skin removed
salt (optional)
freshly ground pepper to taste
1 tablespoon chopped flat-leaf parsley
⅔ cup hot cooked rice
hot pepper sauce for passing

Lightly coat a large pot with cooking spray. Add the okra and cook over medium heat until slightly soft, about 5 minutes. Add the onion, bell peppers, and garlic. Stir, and cook another 5 minutes. Stir in the broth, tomatoes, thyme, cumin, and bay leaf. Simmer, uncovered, for 15 minutes.

Meanwhile, remove the meat from the bone of the chicken thighs. Cut into long strips and discard the bone and any fat. Lightly coat a nonstick skillet with cooking spray. Place over medium-high heat, add the strips of chicken, and cook, turning the strips often, for 5 minutes, or until the chicken is brown and no longer pink in the center (cut to test).

Add the chicken to the okra-tomato mixture and simmer, uncovered, until it is heated through, about 2 to 3 minutes. Taste and adjust the seasoning, adding salt (if using) and pepper. Stir in the parsley and ladle the gumbo into 2 shallow soup bowls. Place half of the hot cooked rice in the center of each serving. Serve at once and pass the hot pepper sauce.

Makes 2 servings.

PER SERVING: 312 calories (18% calories from fat), 6 g total fat (1.5 g saturated fat), 34 g protein, 30 g carbohydrates, 3 g dietary fiber, 118 mg cholesterol, 484 mg sodium

JOSLIN EXCHANGES: 4 very low fat protein, 1 carbohydrate (1 bread/starch), 2 vegetable

Chicken and Mushroom Stew

Ready-to-use frozen stew vegetables make it possible to have this peasant dish prepared in minutes. Add a crusty baguette and a lightly dressed salad of mesclun—a mixture of tiny baby lettuce leaves, savory herbs, edible petals, and wild greens that is sold by the pound or in prepackaged blends in produce markets and some large supermarket chains. You'll think you're dining at a country restaurant in France.

olive oil cooking spray
10 ounces boneless, skinless chicken breast halves, cut into 2-inch strips
½ cup frozen chopped onion
8 ounces button mushrooms
½ cup fat-free reduced-sodium canned chicken broth
2 tablespoons dry white wine or additional chicken broth
2 sprigs fresh thyme or ½ teaspoon crushed dried
1 sprig fresh tarragon or ¼ teaspoon crushed dried
½ bay leaf
1½ cups frozen stew vegetables
1 teaspoon cornstarch
1½ teaspoons lemon juice

Rinse the chicken and pat dry with paper towels. Lightly coat a heavy nonstick skillet with cooking spray. Add the onion, chicken, and mushrooms. Cook over high heat, stirring often, until the chicken begins to brown, about 2 minutes. Lower the heat to medium. Add the broth, wine, herbs, and frozen vegetables.

Stir the cornstarch into the lemon juice until smooth. Add to the skillet and stir until well incorporated. Bring the stew to a simmer, cover, and cook for 15 minutes. Remove the herb sprigs and bay leaf before serving.

Makes 2 servings.

PER SERVING: 278 calories (8% calories from fat), 2 g total fat (0.6 g saturated fat), 38 g protein, 24 g carbohydrates, 3 g dietary fiber, 82 mg cholesterol, 301 mg sodium

JOSLIN EXCHANGES: 4½ very low fat protein, 4 vegetable

Taste the Stew

People often ask how we decide on the amount of spices, salt, pepper, and herbs to use in our recipes. Our response is that we try to match the tastes of the "average" reader, but we hope that you will taste each recipe before serving and modify the seasoning to suit your preference. We also hope you will adjust the herbs and spices that you don't like and substitute others. For example, cilantro, which is used in Mexican and Tex-Mex recipes, may be too strong for you. Some people substitute a small amount of mint for cilantro. Sage is another herb that some people do not like. Thyme is lighter and can be substituted. Pepper, red and black, should be used according to your tolerance for heat.

Please note, however, that we tightly regulate the use of salt in our recipes for medical reasons. Since the complications of diabetes, such as retinopathy, vascular diseases, and heart disease, are linked to hypertension, we limit salt intake. Before adding extra salt, discuss your medical status with your physician and/or health care team.

Easy Turkey Casserole

This casserole can be made ahead up to the point of adding the bread crumbs, then covered and refrigerated. When ready to bake, stir in another ¼ cup of chicken broth, top with the bread crumbs, and bake, adding up to 15 additional minutes to the baking time. ¶ An earthy dish, this is similar to cassoulet—a bean, duck, and sausage combination that is very popular in the south of France.

vegetable cooking spray
2 4-ounce turkey cutlets, cut into thin strips
1 10¼-ounce can fat-free reduced-sodium chicken broth
½ cup frozen chopped onion
1 medium carrot, peeled and cut into ½-inch slices
1 small celery rib with leaves, chopped
1 clove garlic, thinly sliced
1 medium plum tomato, coarsely chopped
½ cup drained canned white beans (Navy or Great Northern)
¼ teaspoon crushed dried thyme
2 tablespoons seasoned bread crumbs (see page 91)

Preheat the oven to 375°F. Lightly coat a shallow 1-quart casserole with cooking spray.

Lightly coat a medium nonstick skillet with cooking spray and place over medium-high heat. Add the turkey pieces and cook, stirring, until the turkey is browned on all sides, about 4 minutes.

In a medium saucepan, bring the broth to a boil. Add the onion, carrot, celery, and garlic. Lower the heat and simmer for 4 minutes. Stir in the turkey pieces, tomato, beans, and thyme. Transfer the mixture to the prepared casserole. Top with the seasoned bread crumbs. Bake, uncovered, until the casserole is browned on the top and bubbling, about 20 minutes.

Makes 2 servings.

PER SERVING: 287 calories (7% calories from fat), 2 g total fat (0.6 g saturated fat), 36 g protein, 33 g carbohydrates, 7 g dietary fiber, 70 mg cholesterol, 622 mg sodium

JOSLIN EXCHANGES: 4 very low fat protein, 1½ carbohydrate (1½ bread/starch), 2 vegetable

Red Beans and Rice

In the South, red beans and rice are almost a religion. Usually cooked from scratch with dried red beans and plenty of bacon fat, the traditional dish is no longer suitable for our lower-fat diets.

This lightened version is mighty good but missing most of the fat. It is based on a recipe given to us by Katherine Cropper, formerly of Atlanta and now living in eastern New Jersey.

5 ounces turkey kielbasa, cut into ½-inch slices
1 medium onion, cut in half, thinly sliced, and separated into rings
1 cup canned red kidney beans, well drained
1 cup canned no-salt-added crushed tomatoes
½ teaspoon Worcestershire sauce
½ teaspoon crushed dried thyme
¼ teaspoon crushed dried sage
¼ teaspoon hot pepper sauce, or to taste
⅔ cup cooked rice
bottle of white vinegar for splashing (optional)

In a heavy-bottomed skillet, brown the turkey kielbasa over medium-high heat, turning frequently, until well browned, about 5 minutes. Transfer to a plate and keep warm. Remove and discard any fat in the skillet.

Add the onion, beans, tomatoes, Worcestershire sauce, thyme, sage, and hot pepper sauce to the skillet and cook over medium heat, stirring often, for 5 minutes. Return the kielbasa to the skillet and add the cooked rice. Cook, stirring, until the rice is heated through, about 5 minutes. Divide the mixture into 2 bowls and pass the bottle of vinegar to sprinkle on the finished dish before eating.

Makes 2 servings.

PER SERVING: 369 calories (16% calories from fat), 7 g total fat (2.0 g saturated fat), 22 g protein, 57 g carbohydrates, 12 g dietary fiber, 47 mg cholesterol, 773 mg sodium

JOSLIN EXCHANGES: 2 low fat protein, 3 carbohydrate (3 bread/starch), 1 vegetable

Southwestern Turkey Meatball Soup

A low-fat version of Albondigas (meatball) soup, this is a hearty low-fat meal-in-a-bowl. We like to float a few crisp strips of corn tortilla and cilantro leaves in the soup at the last minute for color, added flavor, and texture.

vegetable cooking spray
⅓ pound ground white turkey breast
1 small (about 3 ounces) thin-skinned potato, peeled and shredded
1 clove garlic, minced, or ⅛ teaspoon garlic powder
¼ teaspoon ground cumin
2 cups fat-free reduced-sodium canned chicken broth
1 cup fat-free reduced-sodium canned beef broth
1 cup no-salt-added canned tomatoes
½ cup frozen chopped onion
1 small carrot, thinly sliced
1 teaspoon chili powder
¼ teaspoon crushed dried oregano
1 6-inch corn tortilla
1 tablespoon fresh cilantro leaves
1 lime, cut in wedges for squeezing (optional)

Preheat the oven to 500°F. Lightly coat a small baking dish with cooking spray.

In a small bowl, combine the ground turkey, potato, garlic, and cumin. Shape the mixture into 1-inch balls. Place slightly apart in the prepared baking dish and bake for 5 to 7 minutes, until well browned. Using a slotted spatula, remove the turkey balls and drain briefly on paper towels. Lower the oven to 400°F.

Meanwhile, in a large saucepan, bring the broths to a boil over medium-high heat. Coarsely chop the tomatoes and add to the broth along with their juice, the onion, carrot, chili powder, and oregano. Turn the heat to low. Add the turkey balls, partially cover, and simmer for 10 minutes.

While the soup is cooking, cut the corn tortilla into ¼-inch strips. Arrange in a single layer on a baking sheet that has been lightly coated with cooking spray. Bake until crisp, about 10 minutes.

To serve, ladle the soup into 2 shallow soup bowls. Sprinkle each serving with half of the tortilla strips and a few cilantro leaves. Serve with the lime wedges to squeeze into the hot soup if desired.

Makes 2 servings.

PER SERVING: 246 calories (9% calories from fat), 3 g total fat (0.6 g saturated fat), 27 g protein, 31 g carbohydrates, 6 g dietary fiber, 46 mg cholesterol, 709 mg sodium

JOSLIN EXCHANGES: 3 very low fat protein, 1½ carbohydrate (1½ bread/starch), 2 vegetable

Shepherd's Pie, Texas Style

Shepherd's pie usually contains leftover beef and vegetables, but this fresh rendition with a combination of three peppers reflects the boldness of the Texas spirit.

olive oil cooking spray
1 large russet potato, peeled and cut into 2-inch cubes
2 cloves garlic
8 ounces extra-lean ground sirloin
1 small red bell pepper, seeded and diced
1 small yellow bell pepper, seeded and diced
½ cup frozen chopped onion
½ cup frozen corn kernels
2 tablespoons mild or hot salsa
¼ teaspoon crushed dried oregano
2 to 3 tablespoons 1% fat cultured buttermilk
1 tablespoon minced pickled jalapeño slices
½ teaspoon prepared horseradish, or to taste

Preheat the oven to 375°F. Lightly coat a deep 1-quart casserole with cooking spray.

In a medium saucepan, cook the potato and 1 garlic clove in water to cover until tender, about 10 minutes. Drain and transfer to a medium bowl. Cover and keep warm.

Meanwhile, mince the remaining garlic clove. Add to the ground sirloin and cook in a large nonstick skillet over medium-high heat for about 5 minutes, until no longer pink, breaking up the meat with a wooden spoon. Drain off all fat. Add the bell peppers, onion, corn, salsa, and oregano. Cook, stirring, for another 2 minutes. Transfer the mixture to the prepared casserole.

Using a potato masher or electric mixer, mash the potato and garlic until completely smooth. Add the buttermilk as you are mashing. The mixture should have a very soft consistency. Stir in the minced jalapeños and horseradish. Spoon the mixture on the top of the casserole, covering the meat mixture. Smooth the top with the back of a spoon.

Bake, uncovered, for 20 minutes, or until thoroughly heated. Remove from the oven and heat the broiler. Broil 3 inches from heat source for 3 to 4 minutes, until golden brown. Serve at once.

Makes 2 servings.

PER SERVING: 409 calories (21% calories from fat), 10 g total fat (3.7 g saturated fat), 40 g protein, 42 g carbohydrates, 6 g dietary fiber, 102 mg cholesterol, 332 mg sodium

JOSLIN EXCHANGES: 4 low fat protein, 2 carbohydrate (2 bread/starch), 2 vegetable

Sweet-and-Sour Cabbage and Beef Casserole

Here we've modified a favorite stuffed cabbage recipe so it can be ready in minutes, taking advantage of both convenience foods and the microwave. Use the remaining shredded cabbage to make coleslaw for another meal.

vegetable cooking spray
1 cup raw instant rice
8 ounces extra-lean ground sirloin
½ cup frozen chopped onion
1½ tablespoons dark raisins
3 cups shredded cabbage from a 1-pound bag
1 15-ounce can reduced-sodium tomato sauce
1½ tablespoons red wine vinegar
½ teaspoon sugar substitute
freshly ground pepper to taste

Lightly coat a 1-quart microwave-safe casserole dish or 2 individual ramekins with cooking spray.

Cook the instant rice according to the box directions and set aside. Sauté the beef and onion in a large nonstick pan over high heat, breaking up the beef with a wooden spoon until the beef is brown, about 5 minutes. Drain off any fat. Stir in the rice and raisins.

Place the cabbage in a 2-quart microwave-safe casserole. Add 3 tablespoons of water. Cover and cook on HIGH for 2 minutes. Stir and cook for another 1 or 2 minutes, until the cabbage is tender but still crisp to the bite. Drain the cabbage, reserving the cooking liquid.

Add the cabbage cooking liquid to the tomato sauce, along with the vinegar, sugar substitute, and pepper. Stir the sweet-and-sour sauce into the meat and rice mixture.

Place the cooked cabbage on the bottom of the prepared casserole or ramekins. Top with the sweet-and-sour tomato-beef-rice mixture. Cover and microwave on MEDIUM HIGH for 4 minutes. Turn and microwave on MEDIUM HIGH for another 4 minutes. Uncover and allow to sit for 2 minutes before serving.

Makes 2 servings.

PER SERVING: 540 calories (38% calories from fat), 16 g total fat (6.2 g saturated fat), 43 g protein, 72 g carbohydrates, 7 g dietary fiber, 101 mg cholesterol, 154 mg sodium

JOSLIN EXCHANGES: 4 low fat protein, 4 carbohydrate (4 bread/starch), 2 vegetable

Beef and Artichoke Penne Pasta Bake

This recipe makes use of a precooked mixture of ground sirloin, chopped onion, and garlic that we keep in our freezer in easy-to-use 6-ounce portions. The mixture defrosts in the microwave in about 3 minutes, ready for a quick chili, tamale pie, or satisfying casserole. This is a great Sunday night supper dish for eating in front of a roaring fire.

olive oil cooking spray
1 tablespoon grated Parmesan cheese
2 ounces dry penne pasta
1 6-ounce package Beef and Onion Mix (recipe follows), defrosted
4 no-salt-added canned tomatoes, sliced crosswise into quarters
4 canned artichoke hearts, quartered
¾ teaspoon dried mixed Italian herbs
¼ cup juice from no-salt-added canned tomatoes
1 tablespoon tomato paste mixed with 2 tablespoons water
½ cup shredded part-skim milk mozzarella cheese

Preheat the oven to 350°F. Lightly coat a 1-quart casserole or 2 individual au gratin dishes. Sprinkle with the Parmesan cheese.

Cook the pasta according to the package directions for al dente, 10 to 12 minutes. Drain well and add to the defrosted meat mixture. Stir in the tomatoes, artichoke hearts, Italian herbs, tomato juice, and tomato paste with water, mixing gently. Place in the prepared baking dish and sprinkle evenly with the mozzarella cheese. Bake for 20 minutes, or until bubbly hot.

Makes 2 servings.

PER SERVING: 456 calories (28% calories from fat), 14 g total fat (6.4 g saturated fat), 42 g protein, 41 g carbohydrate, 6 g dietary fiber, 94 mg cholesterol, 430 mg sodium

JOSLIN EXCHANGES: 4½ low fat protein, 2 carbohydrate (2 bread/starch), 2 vegetable

Beef and Onion Mix

The microwave is a great way to brown ground meat quickly while extracting most of the fat. This can be done with ground beef, as here, or with ground white meat turkey. The package will then contain 200 calories (9 percent calories from fat), 2 grams total fat, and 104 milligrams of cholesterol.

1½ pounds extra-lean ground sirloin
1 large onion, chopped
4 cloves garlic, minced

Crumble the ground beef into a 3-quart microwave-safe casserole. Cover and cook on HIGH for 5 minutes. Stir to break up the meat. Drain the meat in a colander to remove any fat. Wipe out the microwave dish with paper towels.

Return the beef to the casserole and stir in the onion and garlic. Divide the mixture equally among 4 microwave-safe freezer containers. Cover and freeze. Use within 3 months.

Remove the cover and defrost following your microwave manufacturer's instructions. Use in recipes as needed.

Makes 4 6-ounce packages.

PER PACKAGE: 284 calories (34% calories from fat), 10 g total fat (4.0 g saturated fat), 40 g protein, 6 g carbohydrate, 1 g dietary fiber, 114 mg cholesterol, 86 mg sodium

JOSLIN EXCHANGES: 5½ very low fat protein, 1 vegetable

25-Minute Texas Hill Country Chili

The seasonings in this quick chili are similar to those of the famous Pedernales River Chili that former President Lyndon Baines Johnson made on his ranch in the Texas Hill Country. The use of the precooked Beef and Onion Mix significantly cuts down the cooking time. Note that Texas chili does not contain beans.

1 6-ounce package Beef and Onion Mix (page 173), defrosted
½ to 1 tablespoon good-quality chili powder
¼ teaspoon crushed dried oregano
¼ teaspoon ground cumin
1 14½-ounce can no-salt-added diced tomatoes
1 tablespoon tomato paste
½ cup hot water
salt (optional)

In a heavy saucepan, reheat the Beef and Onion Mix over medium heat, stirring constantly. Add the remaining ingredients except the salt. Bring to a boil. Lower the heat and simmer, uncovered, for 15 to 20 minutes. Skim off and discard any fat that rises to the surface. Taste the chili and add salt (if using). Ladle into 2 soup bowls and serve at once.

Makes 2 servings.

PER SERVING: 197 calories (26% calories from fat), 6 g total fat (2.2 g saturated fat), 22 g protein, 14 g carbohydrates, 5 g dietary fiber, 57 mg cholesterol, 156 mg sodium

JOSLIN EXCHANGES: 3 very low fat protein, 3 vegetable

Italian Beef and Vegetable Skillet Stew

Consider this whole-meal stew when you're hungry and have little time to cook. While the stew is cooking, you can toss a salad of crisp greens. Offer Frozen Grapes (see page 221) for dessert. ⟡ You'll need to purchase a 16-ounce bag of frozen spinach for this dish. Since you'll be using only ½ cup for this recipe, there will be plenty of spinach left for one or two meals. Another time, substitute chopped broccoli.

2 ounces elbow macaroni
1 6-ounce package Beef and Onion Mix (page 173), defrosted
1 cup canned no-salt-added tomatoes, drained
2 tablespoons tomato paste

½ cup reduced-sodium vegetable juice
½ teaspoon crushed dried basil
½ teaspoon crushed dried oregano
½ cup frozen chopped spinach
salt (optional)
freshly ground pepper
3 tablespoons shredded skim-milk mozzarella cheese
thinly sliced scallions for garnish (optional)

Bring a medium pot of water to a rapid boil. Add the macaroni and cook according to package directions to al dente, about 10 minutes.

Meanwhile, place the Beef and Onion Mix in a heavy nonstick skillet over medium heat. Coarsely chop the tomatoes and add to the meat mixture with their juice. Stir in the tomato paste, vegetable juice, basil, and oregano. Lower the heat, cover, and simmer for 5 minutes. Stir in the spinach. Cook, uncovered, until the spinach is just wilted, stirring frequently.

Drain the cooked macaroni and stir into the meat-vegetable mixture. Cover and continue to simmer for another 5 minutes. Taste and adjust the seasoning, adding salt (if using) and pepper to taste. Sprinkle with the cheese. Cover and continue to cook until the cheese melts, about 3 minutes.

To serve, spoon the stew onto 2 dinner plates and garnish with sliced scallions if desired. Serve at once.

Makes 3 servings.

PER SERVING: 340 calories (21% calories from fat), 8 g total fat (3.3 g saturated fat), 30 g protein, 38 g carbohydrates, 6 g dietary fiber, 62 mg cholesterol, 293 mg sodium

JOSLIN EXCHANGES: 3 very low fat protein, 1½ carbohydrate (1½ bread/starch), 3 vegetable

Meatless White Chili

This spicy white chili has no meat; it gets its protein from the beans. If you wish, poach a 5-ounce chicken breast in the microwave, then shred it and add it to the chili during the last 5 minutes of cooking time. Adding chicken will increase each serving by 78 calories, 1 gram of fat, 16 grams of protein, and 2 very low fat protein exchanges.

1 teaspoon canola oil
½ cup frozen chopped onion
2 tablespoons minced celery leaves
1 clove garlic, minced
½ jalapeño chile pepper, seeded and minced
½ teaspoon ground cumin
½ teaspoon crushed dried oregano
⅛ teaspoon crushed dried thyme
pinch cayenne pepper
pinch ground cloves
2 cups plus up to ¼ cup low-sodium canned chicken or vegetable broth, defatted
1 15-ounce can Great Northern beans, rinsed and well drained
1 tablespoon minced fresh cilantro
1 tablespoon minced flat-leaf parsley
salt (optional)
freshly ground pepper to taste

Condiments:

2 tablespoons minced fresh cilantro
2 tablespoons minced red onion
2 tablespoons fat-free sour cream

In a large nonstick saucepan, heat the oil over low heat. Add the onion, celery leaves, garlic, and jalapeño. Cook, stirring, until the onion is soft, about 4 minutes. (Do not let the onion or garlic brown.) Stir in the cumin, oregano, thyme, cayenne pepper, and cloves.

Gradually add 2 cups of the chicken broth, stirring constantly. Stir in the beans, cilantro, and parsley. Cover and simmer for 15 minutes, stirring occasionally.

Taste the chili and add salt (if using) and pepper to taste. If the chili is too thick, stir in the additional ¼ cup of chicken broth, 1 tablespoon at a time, until the desired consistency is reached (chili should be thick).

Ladle the chili into two soup bowls. Place the condiments in small individual bowls and serve with the chili, to be spooned on each serving.

Makes 2 servings.

PER SERVING: 278 calories (11% calories from fat), 3 g total fat (0.8 g saturated fat), 20 g protein, 47 g carbohydrates, 12 g dietary fiber, 6 mg cholesterol, 565 mg sodium

JOSLIN EXCHANGES: 1½ very low fat protein, 3½ carbohydrate (3½ bread/starch)

Curried Tofu and Vegetables

Tofu or soybean curd is a good source of calcium and is recommended to those who are allergic to dairy products. It's high in protein, low in calories, low in fat, low in sodium and cholesterol free—and it's also inexpensive. The chameleon of foods, it takes on the flavors of the other ingredients it is cooked with, such as the curry and other aromatic spices here. Using frozen vegetables, this savory dish will be on the table in minutes. Serve it over bowls of steamed basmati or brown rice. ❡ You'll need to press the tofu (see below) before you stir-fry it. This makes the cooking easier and removes unwanted liquid from the tofu.

6 ounces firm tofu, drained and pressed
vegetable cooking spray
1 clove garlic, minced
1 tablespoon minced fresh ginger
¾ teaspoon curry powder (for hot curry; decrease to ½ teaspoon for moderate)
⅛ teaspoon ground cinnamon
⅛ teaspoon ground cumin
⅓ cup frozen chopped onion
1 small tomato, seeded and chopped
1 tablespoon water
2 cups frozen vegetable medley (broccoli, cauliflower, and carrots)
¼ cup plain nonfat yogurt
2 teaspoons currants or golden raisins

Press the tofu: Wrap it in a double layer of paper towels, place on a plate, and top with a heavy pan or dish. Set aside.

Meanwhile, lightly coat a nonstick skillet with cooking spray. Add the garlic, ginger, curry, cinnamon, and cumin. Stir over medium heat for 30 seconds to release the aromas. Add the onion and stir-fry for 1 minute, until the onion is thawed. Add the tomato and water. Continue to stir-fry for 2 minutes.

Remove the paper towels from the tofu and slice it into ½-inch slices. Add the tofu to the skillet, cover, and simmer for 10 minutes. Stir in the frozen vegetables, cover, and cook until the vegetables are warmed through but still crisp, about 4 minutes. Remove from the heat and gently stir in the yogurt and currants. Serve at once.

Makes 2 servings.

PER SERVING: 222 calories (29% calories from fat), 8 g total fat (1.2 g saturated fat), 20 g protein, 24 g carbohydrates, 6 g dietary fiber, 1 mg cholesterol, 97 mg sodium

JOSLIN EXCHANGES: 2 medium fat protein, 4 vegetable

Lentils and Brown Rice with Tofu

This recipe comes from Parvine Latimore, a Persian friend from Westport, Connecticut, and a gifted cook who now specializes in vegetarian dishes. ❡ The lentils and brown rice must be cooked separately, so it's best to cook them the night before or early that morning. Then the finished dish goes together in a matter of minutes.

1 teaspoon olive oil
1 cup frozen chopped onion
½ cup frozen chopped green bell pepper
4 ounces firm tofu, pressed (see page 177) and cut into 1-inch cubes
½ cup cooked lentils
½ cup cooked brown rice
1 tablespoon reduced-sodium soy sauce
juice of ½ fresh lime

In a heavy-bottomed skillet, heat the oil over medium-high heat. Add the onion and bell pepper. Cook, stirring, until the onion is lightly browned, about 5 minutes. Add the tofu and continue to stir-fry for another 2 minutes, until the tofu is lightly browned. Add the remaining ingredients and cook, stirring gently, for another 2 to 3 minutes, until the lentils and rice are heated through. Serve at once.

Makes 2 servings.

PER SERVING: 258 calories (26% calories from fat), 8 g total fat (1.2 g saturated fat), 16 g protein, 34 g carbohydrates, 5 g dietary fiber, 0 cholesterol, 276 mg sodium

JOSLIN EXCHANGES: 1½ medium fat protein, 1½ carbohydrate (1½ bread/starch), 1 vegetable

{ Grains and Other Starches }

Crispy Garlic Potatoes

Excellent with grilled meat and fish, these potatoes will fill your craving for fat-laden French fries.

olive oil cooking spray
2 small russet potatoes (about 8 ounces total), scrubbed
1 tablespoon olive oil
1 teaspoon crushed dried rosemary
¼ teaspoon garlic powder

Preheat the oven to 475°F. Lightly coat a large nonstick baking sheet with cooking spray.

Using a sharp knife, cut the potatoes into quarters lengthwise. Cut each quarter into ¼-inch slices. Place the potato slices in a single layer on the baking sheet. Drizzle with oil, turning to coat evenly. Sprinkle with rosemary and garlic powder. Lightly coat the potatoes with cooking spray. Bake for 15 minutes, turning once, to brown evenly.

Remove from the oven and transfer the potato slices to a paper towel to absorb any excess oil. Serve immediately.

Makes 2 servings.

PER SERVING: 186 calories (33% calories from fat), 7 g total fat (0.9 g saturated fat), 3 g protein, 29 g carbohydrates, 3 g dietary fiber, 0 cholesterol, 9 mg sodium

JOSLIN EXCHANGES: 2 carbohydrate (2 bread/starch), 1 fat

Red Potato Salad

The addition of the cucumber here gives each bite a lovely combination of textures. All you need are hot coals in your barbecue to make this summertime favorite part of a lazy afternoon or evening.

8 ounces whole small red or white potatoes, or larger potatoes cut in half or quartered, washed, skin left on
6 ounces of cucumber, peeled, halved, seeded, and thinly sliced

Dressing:

2½ tablespoons fat-free sour cream
1 tablespoon reduced-calorie mayonnaise
1 tablespoon white wine vinegar
½ teaspoon Dijon mustard
⅛ teaspoon celery seeds
⅛ teaspoon onion powder
⅛ teaspoon garlic powder
freshly ground pepper to taste

Boil the potatoes in lightly salted water until cooked through, about 10 minutes. Test with the sharp point of a knife. Drain and cool until you can handle them. If using small creamers, slice in half; slice larger potatoes in quarters. Place in a bowl and add the cucumber.

In a cup or small bowl, combine the sour cream with the remaining dressing ingredients. Toss with the potatoes and cucumber.

Makes 2 servings.

PER SERVING: 178 calories (9% calories from fat), 2 g total fat (0.3 g saturated fat), 4 g protein, 36 g carbohydrates, 3 g dietary fiber, 2 mg cholesterol, 96 mg sodium

JOSLIN EXCHANGES: 2 carbohydrate (2 bread/starch), 1 vegetable

Garlic Mashed Potatoes

Baby new potatoes are available from early spring to late summer and make the most satisfying mashed potatoes. Buy small amounts and use them quickly, for once they're out of the ground, their natural sugars begin to turn to starch and they begin to lose their vitamins. At other times of the year, use peeled thin-skinned white potatoes or peeled or unpeeled Yukon Gold potatoes. ❡ In this recipe you can choose to add prepared horseradish or minced pickled jalapeño chiles. Add one or both, or leave the potatoes plain. In any way, they're delicious.

8 ounces baby potatoes, scrubbed
2 cloves garlic, peeled and cut in half
about ⅓ cup skim milk, heated
1 teaspoon prepared horseradish or to taste (optional)
1 teaspoon minced pickled jalapeño chiles (optional)
salt (optional)
freshly ground pepper to taste

If the potatoes are about 1 inch in diameter, leave them whole. If large, cut in half or quarter them. Drop into a pot of boiling water along with the garlic.

Lower the heat to medium and boil until the potatoes are tender, about 10 minutes. Drain off the water and return the potatoes and garlic to the pot. Shake over the heat for 1 minute to remove the remaining moisture.

Begin mashing the potatoes with a potato masher or electric mixer. Add the hot milk gradually, until the mixture is smooth and fluffy with no lumps. If desired, whip in the horseradish, minced jalapeño, or both. Taste and season with salt (if using) and pepper to taste. Serve immediately.

Makes 2 servings.

PER SERVING: 142 calories (1% calories from fat), <1 g total fat (trace saturated fat), 4 g protein, 32 g carbohydrates, 3 g dietary fiber, 1 mg cholesterol, 31 mg sodium

JOSLIN EXCHANGES: 2 carbohydrate (2 bread/starch)

Medley of Winter Roots

Years ago we fell in love with a similar recipe in Martha Stewart's *Quick Cook*, but unfortunately that dish was loaded with butter. In this version the vegetables are steamed and then tossed with a single teaspoon of olive oil—just enough to allow the thyme to adhere. No need for another drop.

> 1 very small sweet potato, peeled and cut into 1-inch cubes
> 1 very small thin-skinned white potato, scrubbed and cut into 1-inch cubes
> 1 small carrot, scrubbed and cut into 1-inch cubes
> 1 very small turnip, peeled and cut into 1-inch cubes
> 1 teaspoon olive oil
> ½ teaspoon minced fresh thyme or ⅛ teaspoon crushed dried
> salt (optional)
> freshly ground pepper to taste

In a vegetable steamer or colander placed over simmering water, steam the vegetables until just tender, about 10 to 12 minutes. Drizzle the vegetables with the olive oil and toss with the thyme, salt (if using), and pepper. Serve at once.

Makes 2 servings.

PER SERVING: 141 calories (16% calories from fat), 3 g total fat (0.4 g saturated fat), 2 g protein, 28 g carbohydrates, 4 g dietary fiber, 0 cholesterol, 52 mg sodium

JOSLIN EXCHANGES: 1 carbohydrate (1 bread/starch), 2 vegetable

Cajun Spiced Rice

Cajun cooking brings thoughts of southern Louisiana, spices, jazz, and good food. This recipe for rice makes a tasty side dish, but adding spiced shrimp, seafood, and a bit of spiced turkey sausage makes it an entire meal. Its pungent, aromatic mixture of spices and herbs is typical of Cajun cooking. Pass the hot sauce, please.

> butter-flavored cooking spray
> ½ cup frozen chopped onion
> 1 small green bell pepper, chopped
> 1 tablespoon celery flakes
> 1 cup low-sodium canned chicken broth
> 1 cup raw instant rice
> 1 clove garlic, minced, or ⅛ teaspoon garlic powder
> ⅛ teaspoon crushed dried basil

⅛ teaspoon freshly ground black pepper
⅛ teaspoon cayenne pepper, or to taste
⅛ teaspoon crushed dried thyme

Lightly coat a medium nonstick saucepan with cooking spray. Add the onion, bell pepper, and celery flakes. Cook over medium-high heat, stirring occasionally, until the onion wilts, about 4 minutes.

Add the broth, rice, garlic, basil, black pepper, cayenne pepper, and thyme. Bring to a boil, cover, and remove from the heat. Let stand for 5 minutes. Fluff with a fork and serve.

Makes 2 servings.

PER SERVING: 217 calories (2% calories from fat), 1 g total fat (0.1 g saturated fat), 5 g protein, 48 g carbohydrates, 3 g dietary fiber, 0 cholesterol, 66 mg sodium

JOSLIN EXCHANGES: 3 carbohydrate (3 bread/starch)

Mediterranean Spiced Rice

This rice with North African flavorings is perfect with grilled chicken or fish. Another time, make a double batch for a great company salad, dressed with a splash of Lemon-Balsamic Dressing (page 203).

butter-flavored cooking spray
¼ cup frozen chopped onion
2 cloves garlic, minced, or ¼ teaspoon garlic powder
1 cup water
1 cup raw instant rice
¼ cup shredded carrot
1 teaspoon grated lemon zest
¼ teaspoon ground cumin
⅛ teaspoon cayenne pepper (optional)
⅛ teaspoon ground cinnamon
⅛ teaspoon salt (optional)
½ teaspoon lemon juice

Lightly coat a medium nonstick saucepan with cooking spray. Add the onion and garlic. Sauté over medium heat until the onion wilts, about 4 minutes. Add the water and bring to a boil. Stir in the rice, carrot, lemon zest, cumin, cayenne pepper (if using), cinnamon, salt (if using), and lemon juice.

Cover and remove from the heat. Let stand for 5 minutes. Fluff with a fork and serve.

Makes 2 servings.

PER SERVING: 200 calories (1% calories from fat), <1 g total fat (trace saturated fat), 4 g protein, 44 g carbohydrates, 2 g dietary fiber, 0 cholesterol, 12 mg sodium

JOSLIN EXCHANGES: 3 carbohydrate (3 bread/starch)

Dilled Rice with Baby Peas

Rice and baby peas are a classic combination. Here we marry them with fresh dill, which gives them a summer taste all year long. ❡ The recipe can also serve as the basis for a salad by adding leftover cooked vegetables and serving on a bed of lettuce that has been dressed with a light lemon-based vinaigrette using the ratio of one part lemon juice to two parts nonfat plain yogurt, seasoned with pepper and dill. You can figure your extra exchanges using the Joslin Exchanges (page 249).

> *½ cup low-sodium canned chicken broth*
> *½ cup water*
> *½ cup frozen baby peas*
> *1 tablespoon chopped fresh dill or 1 teaspoon dried dill weed*
> *1 cup raw instant rice*
> *freshly ground pepper to taste*

Place the broth and water in a saucepan with a cover and bring to a boil. Meanwhile, place the peas in a microwave-safe bowl and cover. Microwave on DEFROST for 1 minute.

When the broth and water is boiling, stir in the peas, dill, and rice. Cover and set aside for 5 minutes. Add the pepper. Fluff with a fork and serve.

Makes 2 servings.

PER SERVING: 216 calories (3% calories from fat), 1 g total fat (0.3 g saturated fat), 6 g protein, 45 g carbohydrates, 3 g dietary fiber, 1 mg cholesterol, 72 mg sodium

JOSLIN EXCHANGES: 3 carbohydrate (3 bread/starch)

Lemon Rice with Dried Apricots

Fruit and rice make an excellent accompaniment for plain grilled meats and poultry. Try your favorite dried fruit, making sure to keep the exchanges the same as in this recipe (see Joslin Exchanges, page 255).

½ cup low-sodium canned chicken broth
½ cup water
1 teaspoon grated lemon zest
1 clove garlic, minced, or ⅛ teaspoon garlic powder
1 cup raw instant rice
¼ cup chopped dried apricots (about 8)
freshly ground pepper to taste

Place the broth and water in a saucepan with a cover and bring to a boil. Add the lemon zest, garlic, and rice. Cover, remove from the heat, and let stand for 5 minutes. Add the apricots and pepper, fluffing with a fork. Serve at once.

Makes 2 servings.

PER SERVING: 255 calories (2% calories from fat), 1 g total fat (0.3 g saturated fat), 6 g protein, 58 g carbohydrates, 1 g dietary fiber, 1 mg cholesterol, 33 mg sodium

JOSLIN EXCHANGES: 4 carbohydrate (3 bread/starch, 1 fruit)

Easy Fried Rice

Usually loaded with oil, this lightened version of fried rice uses only a teaspoon. With all its flavor, you won't miss the fat. You'll need to make the rice ahead—maybe earlier in the week. It'll keep for several days in the refrigerator. ❡ You can include bits of cooked fish or chicken when you add the rice to make this a whole meal. Check with the Joslin Exchanges (page 264) for your additional exchanges.

½ teaspoon canola oil
½ teaspoon dark sesame oil
1 tablespoon minced fresh ginger
1 shallot, minced, or 1 tablespoon minced red onion
1 clove garlic, minced
1 cup coarsely chopped Chinese (napa) cabbage
⅓ cup frozen mixed vegetables
1 cup cooked white rice
1 tablespoon reduced-sodium soy sauce
1 tablespoon dry sherry
1 large egg white, slightly beaten

In a large nonstick skillet, heat both oils over medium heat. Add the ginger, shallot, and garlic. Cook, stirring frequently, until the shallot wilts, about 4 minutes. Do not let the shallot or garlic get too brown.

Raise the heat to medium-high. Add the cabbage and mixed vegetables. Stir-fry for 4 minutes. Add the rice, soy sauce, and sherry. Continue to stir-fry until the rice is hot, about 1 minute. Make a well in the center of the rice-vegetable mixture and add the egg white. Fold into the rice-vegetable mixture and cook for another minute. Serve at once.

Makes 2 servings.

PER SERVING: 207 calories (13% calories from fat), 3 g total fat (0.3 g saturated fat), 7 g protein, 37 g carbohydrates, 2 g dietary fiber, 0 cholesterol, 324 mg sodium

JOSLIN EXCHANGES: 2 carbohydrate (2 bread/starch), 1 vegetable

Couscous with Currants and Walnuts

Couscous is a staple of the people from northern Africa. It is flour-coated semolina, the same ground durum wheat used to make the flour for pasta.

½ teaspoon ground cinnamon
½ teaspoon ground cumin
1 tablespoon dried currants
1 teaspoon reduced-calorie margarine
⅔ cup instant couscous
3 tablespoons chopped fresh parsley
½ teaspoon crushed dried thyme
½ tablespoon chopped walnuts

Place 1 cup of water in a pot with a cover. Add the cinnamon, cumin, currants, and margarine, and bring to a boil. Stir in the couscous, parsley, and thyme. Cover the pot, remove from the heat, and let stand for 5 minutes. Fluff with a fork and sprinkle with the walnuts. Serve immediately.

Makes 2 servings.

PER SERVING: 257 calories (14% calories from fat), 4 g total fat (0.2 g saturated fat), 9 g protein, 50 g carbohydrates, 3 g dietary fiber, 0 cholesterol, 18 mg sodium

JOSLIN EXCHANGES: 3 carbohydrate (3 bread/starch)

Kasha with Zucchini

If you grew up in a family whose origins were eastern European, you know a dish with kasha (buckwheat groats) and bow ties. Here is a slightly different but equally delicious version that complements beef and chicken.

butter-flavored cooking spray
¼ cup frozen chopped onion
2 small zucchini (about 6 ounces total), sliced into 1-inch-long matchsticks
½ cup raw kasha
1 cup low-sodium canned chicken broth
freshly ground pepper to taste

Lightly coat a large nonstick skillet with cooking spray. Add the onion and zucchini, and sauté over medium-high heat until almost tender, about 3 minutes. Transfer to a plate.

Add the kasha to the pan and sauté over high heat to toast for 2 to 3 minutes. Lower the heat to medium. Add the broth, reserved vegetables, and pepper. Bring to a simmer, cover, and cook until the liquid has been absorbed, about 15 minutes. Fluff with a fork before serving.

Makes 2 servings.

PER SERVING: 202 calories (18% calories from fat), 4 g total fat (0.5 g saturated fat), 9 g protein, 35 g carbohydrates, 7 g dietary fiber, 2 mg cholesterol, 76 mg sodium

JOSLIN EXCHANGES: 2 carbohydrate (2 bread/starch), 1 vegetable

Corn Pudding

This is a lightened version of an old-fashioned dish. You'll need two 6-ounce ramekins or soufflé dishes for this recipe.

vegetable cooking spray
1 cup fresh or frozen corn kernels
1 large egg white
¼ cup 1% fat cultured buttermilk
1 tablespoon minced onion
1 tablespoon minced red bell pepper
⅛ teaspoon dry mustard
⅛ teaspoon Worcestershire sauce
1 tablespoon reduced-fat sharp cheddar cheese
⅛ teaspoon salt (optional)
freshly ground pepper to taste

Preheat the oven to 375°F. Lightly coat two 6-ounce ramekins with cooking spray.

In a food processor or blender, combine ½ cup of the corn with the egg white and buttermilk. Process until smooth. Transfer the mixture to a small bowl and add the remaining ½ cup of corn, onion, bell pepper, mustard, Worcestershire sauce, cheese, salt (if using), and pepper.

Divide the mixture between the 2 prepared ramekins. Bake for 20 to 25 minutes, until puffed and set in the center. Serve warm.

Makes 2 servings.

PER SERVING: 106 calories (17% calories from fat), 2 g total fat (0.8 g saturated fat), 7 g protein, 17 g carbohydrates, 2 g dietary fiber, 4 mg cholesterol, 102 mg sodium

JOSLIN EXCHANGES: ½ low fat protein, 1 carbohydrate (1 bread/starch)

Broiled Polenta with Tomatoes and Peppers

Polenta, which is made of corn, is northern Italian and is eaten soft or firm. The latter is cut into slices and grilled or fried. In Italy it's usually eaten for breakfast or dinner. Nowadays you can buy polenta already cooked and formed in 1-pound-roll packages in the produce section of your grocery store. Or you can prepare instant polenta following the package directions. Spread the cooked polenta in a shallow baking dish, cool, and cut into squares.

Tomato and pepper topping:

¼ cup frozen chopped onion
1 clove garlic, minced, or ⅛ teaspoon garlic powder
1 14½-ounce can no-salt-added diced tomatoes, drained well
1 medium red bell pepper, sliced into thin strips
1 medium green bell pepper, sliced into thin strips
4 ounces button mushrooms, thinly sliced
1 tablespoon chopped fresh basil or 1 teaspoon crushed dried
freshly ground pepper to taste

8 ounces prepared nonfat polenta, Italian herb variety, cut into 4 slices
butter-flavored cooking spray

Preheat the broiler.

In a large nonstick skillet, sauté the onion and garlic over medium-high heat until the onion is wilted, about 4 minutes. Add the remaining topping ingredients. Cook over high heat, stirring frequently, for 3 to 5 minutes, until the vegetables are tender. Keep warm.

Lightly coat the broiler pan with cooking spray. Place the polenta slices on the broiler pan and broil 4 to 5 inches from the heat source for 3 minutes per side, until brown on both sides. Coat again with cooking spray after turning once.

Place the grilled polenta on dinner plates. Top with the vegetables and sauce. Serve immediately.

Makes 2 servings.

PER SERVING: 192 calories (5% calories from fat), 1 g total fat (trace saturated fat), 7 g protein, 42 g carbohydrates, 9 g dietary fiber, 0 cholesterol, 392 mg sodium

JOSLIN EXCHANGES: 2 carbohydrate (2 bread/starch), 2 vegetable

Simply Delicious Black Beans

Serve these terrific black beans with grilled chicken or fish. They are pleasingly spiced and very easy to make.

2 tablespoons chopped red onion
1 teaspoon olive oil
1 15-ounce can black beans, drained
1 tablespoon balsamic vinegar
1 tablespoon fresh lemon juice
¼ teaspoon ground cumin
¼ teaspoon crushed dried oregano
dash cayenne pepper
1 tablespoon minced fresh cilantro or flat-leaf parsley

In a medium nonstick saucepan, sauté the red onion in olive oil over low heat until the onion wilts, about 4 minutes. Stir in the drained beans, vinegar, lemon juice, cumin, oregano, and cayenne pepper. Simmer, uncovered, for 5 minutes, stirring occasionally. If the beans seem too dry, add 1 to 2 tablespoons of water. Stir in the cilantro. Serve hot.

Makes 2 servings.

PER SERVING: 202 calories (17% calories from fat), 4 g total fat (0.3 g saturated fat), 12 g protein, 32 g carbohydrates, 12 g dietary fiber, 0 cholesterol, 656 mg sodium

JOSLIN EXCHANGES: 1 very low fat protein, 2 carbohydrate (2 bread/starch)

Spinach with Garbanzo Beans

The cooks of Seville in the south of Spain have a particularly wonderful talent when it comes to preparing vegetables. This Andalusian treatment of fresh spinach is an excellent example—a simple combination that sings. This vegetable dish is frequently served aboard cruise ships sailing in the western Mediterranean.

2 teaspoons olive oil
1 clove garlic, minced
¼ cup chopped red bell pepper
1 pound fresh spinach, well washed and large stems removed
½ cup canned garbanzo beans (chickpeas), well drained, rinsed, and drained again
salt (optional)
freshly ground pepper to taste

In a large heavy-bottomed skillet, heat the olive oil and add the garlic and bell pepper. Sauté over low heat until the garlic is lightly browned and the bell pepper is soft, about 5 minutes. Add the spinach and cook, stirring, just until the spinach wilts. Add the garbanzo beans. Season with salt (if using) and pepper. Continue to cook until the garbanzo beans are heated through. Serve at once.

Makes 2 servings.

PER SERVING: 148 calories (33% calories from fat), 6 g total fat (0.8 g saturated fat), 10 g protein, 18 g carbohydrates, 9 g dietary fiber, 0 cholesterol, 291 mg sodium

JOSLIN EXCHANGES: ½ very low fat protein, 1 carbohydrate (1 bread/starch), 1 vegetable, 1 fat

{ Vegetables and Salads }

Grilled Vegetable Skewers

If fresh corn isn't in season, you can use frozen corn on the cob. The grilling brings out the corn's natural sugars and gives it a fresh-picked flavor. The other vegetables are available year-round.

1 teaspoon chopped fresh basil or ¼ teaspoon crushed dried
1 teaspoon chopped fresh rosemary or ¼ teaspoon crushed dried
1 teaspoon chopped fresh thyme or ¼ teaspoon dried
1 clove garlic, finely minced, or ⅛ teaspoon garlic powder
⅛ teaspoon salt (optional)
freshly ground pepper to taste
1 medium ear of corn, husk removed (if frozen, thaw for a few minutes under cold running water)
1 small zucchini, ends trimmed
4 large cherry tomatoes
¼ small red onion, peeled and cut in half
olive oil cooking spray

Start a charcoal or gas grill.

In a small bowl, combine the basil, rosemary, thyme, garlic, salt (if using), and pepper.

Cut the corn and zucchini into 4 even pieces. Thread the vegetables on two 8-inch skewers in this order: a piece of corn, tomato, zucchini, onion, zucchini, tomato, corn. Lightly coat on all sides with cooking spray and sprinkle with the basil-herb mixture.

Grill the skewers over medium-hot heat, 4 to 6 inches from the heat source, for 5 minutes on each of 4 sides, or until the vegetables are cooked through. Serve immediately.

Makes 2 servings.

PER SERVING: 78 calories (10% calories from fat), 1 g total fat (0.2 g saturated fat), 3 g protein, 17 g carbohydrates, 3 g dietary fiber, 0 cholesterol, 15 mg sodium

JOSLIN EXCHANGES: ½ carbohydrate (½ bread/starch), 1 vegetable

Grilling Vegetables

Grilling or barbecuing knows no season. We've always been wild about the charred flavor of grilled food, and that's particularly true of vegetables.

Some vegetables, such as whole potatoes and corn on the cob, can be wrapped in foil and placed on the coals of the barbecue. Soft vegetables can be cooked on foil so they don't fall into the coals. Larger vegetables can be placed in wire baskets so they are easier to turn. To hasten their cooking time, root vegetables, such as potatoes, carrots, beets, and fennel, should be parboiled on the stove before being placed on the grill. All vegetables to be grilled need to be spritzed with flavored cooking spray so they remain moist.

In addition to charcoal, try experimenting with different woods: Fruitwoods (apple, cherry, peach, pear, apricot, citrus), oak, hickory, mesquite, and sprigs of pine can all be used to add an exciting flavor. Grapevines and the dried stalks of last summer's sweet basil are the latest additions to the grilling craze. They burn very hot and impart a light smokiness. You can also place bundles of fresh herbs on the coals to produce a great flavor. Experiment and enjoy the new flavors.

Broiled Tomatoes with Feta Cheese

This is a simple and quick vegetable dish to serve alongside grilled meats and chicken. Another time, use shredded part-skim mozzarella cheese in place of the feta, and oregano instead of dill.

olive oil cooking spray
2 medium-firm ripe tomatoes
2 tablespoons crumbled feta cheese
2 teaspoons minced fresh dill or ½ teaspoon dried dill weed
freshly ground pepper

Preheat the broiler. Lightly coat a small baking pan with cooking spray.

Slice each tomato crosswise into 3 slices. Arrange, cut side up, in a single layer in the prepared baking pan. Sprinkle with feta cheese and dill. Spritz the cooking spray over the top and season with pepper.

Broil until the cheese melts and starts to brown, about 7 minutes. Serve at once.

Makes 2 servings.

PER SERVING: 49 calories (34% calories from fat), 2 g total fat (1.3 g saturated fat), 2 g protein, 6 g carbohydrates, 1 g dietary fiber, 6 mg cholesterol, 88 mg sodium

JOSLIN EXCHANGE: 1 vegetable

Baked Asparagus with Lemon Bread Crumbs

This is one of our favorite ways to prepare fresh asparagus. Baking or roasting any vegetable intensifies its flavor, and we particularly like what it does to asparagus. As the spears brown, they become crunchy, and when tossed with the lemony bread crumbs, they are simple perfection.

butter-flavored cooking spray
8 ounces fresh asparagus, woody stems snapped off and discarded
1½ tablespoons fine fresh bread crumbs
1 teaspoon grated lemon zest
½ tablespoon fresh lemon juice
freshly ground pepper
1 clove garlic, minced, or ⅛ teaspoon garlic powder (optional)

Preheat the oven to 450°F. Lightly coat a shallow nonstick baking pan with cooking spray.

Place the asparagus in a single layer in the pan. Turn each spear to coat all sides with the cooking spray. Bake until tender but still crisp, 8 to 10 minutes, turning each spear once.

Meanwhile, combine the remaining ingredients and toast on a small baking sheet for 1 to 2 minutes in a toaster oven (or a 375° oven) until golden brown. Stir once to ensure even toasting.

Place the baked asparagus on a serving plate and sprinkle with the lemon bread crumbs.

Makes 2 servings.

PER SERVING: 48 calories (8% calories from fat), < 1 g total fat (0.1 g saturated fat), 3 g protein, 10 g carbohydrates, 3 g dietary fiber, 0 cholesterol, 43 mg sodium

JOSLIN EXCHANGES: 2 vegetable

Baked Ratatouille

This popular vegetable dish owes its origin to Provence. The ingredients can either be cooked together or, as in our recipe, separately in the oven to intensify their flavors. Since several vegetables are used, there will be ample ratatouille left over for another meal. Actually, the flavor improves with age, so it'll be delicious served cold, warm, or hot the second day.

12 ounces eggplant, peeled and cut into ⅓-inch slices
½ teaspoon salt (optional)
2 small zucchini (8 ounces total), washed and cut into ½-inch slices
1 small (4 ounces) onion, peeled and cut into ¼-inch slices
3 plum tomatoes (8 ounces total), cut into thirds lengthwise
1 medium (6 ounces) green bell pepper, seeded and cut into 6 pieces lengthwise
olive oil cooking spray
freshly ground pepper to taste
1 clove garlic, minced, or ⅛ teaspoon garlic powder
2 tablespoons chopped fresh basil or ¾ teaspoon crushed dried

Preheat the oven to 475°F.

While the oven is heating, sprinkle the cut eggplant with salt (if using) and let stand while preparing the remaining vegetables. When ready to cook, use a damp paper towel to remove all visible salt from the eggplant. (Even this quick salting will improve the taste of the eggplant.)

Lightly coat a nonstick cookie sheet with cooking spray and arrange the vegetables on it in a single layer. Sprinkle pepper on top and coat the vegetables with cooking spray. Bake for 15 minutes.

Remove the vegetables from the oven and place in a heavy pot with a cover. Add the garlic and basil, cover, bring to a simmer, and cook for 5 to 8 minutes, until the individual flavors meld.

Serve as a side dish for grilled meats and poultry or as a topping for baked potato, polenta, rice, or pasta.

Makes 4 servings.

PER SERVING: 68 calories (6% calories from fat), 1 g total fat (0.1 g saturated fat), 3 g protein, 16 g carbohydrates, 5 g dietary fiber, 0 cholesterol, 11 mg sodium

JOSLIN EXCHANGES: 3 vegetable

Roasted Cauliflower Parmesan

Cauliflower is high in vitamin C, folic acid (a B vitamin), and fiber. It is also included on the list of antioxidant vegetables—the vegetables associated with reduced cancer rates when eaten regularly. Finding new ways to enjoy cauliflower is therefore a bonus for our diets. Here is one that will satisfy both you and your need for vegetables.

olive oil cooking spray
½ tablespoon olive oil
½ tablespoon lemon juice
⅛ teaspoon kosher salt (optional)
freshly ground pepper to taste
½ head cauliflower (about 14 ounces), broken into florets
½ tablespoon fine fresh bread crumbs
1 tablespoon grated Parmesan cheese

Preheat the oven to 475°F. Lightly coat a shallow nonstick baking pan with cooking spray.

In a large bowl, whisk together the olive oil, lemon juice, salt (if using), and pepper. Add the cauliflower florets and lightly toss to coat evenly. Transfer the cauliflower to the baking pan and drizzle with any olive oil mixture left in bowl. Roast for 12 to 15 minutes, until browned and just tender. Turn the florets once while roasting.

Meanwhile, lightly toast the bread crumbs in a toaster oven (or 275° oven). Combine with the cheese. When the cauliflower is done, top with the bread crumb mixture. Serve hot or at room temperature.

Makes 2 servings.

PER SERVING: 101 calories (38% calories from fat), 5 g total fat (1.1 g saturated fat), 5 g protein, 12 g carbohydrates, 4 g dietary fiber, 2 mg cholesterol, 131 mg sodium

JOSLIN EXCHANGES: 2 vegetable, 1 fat

The Fruit of the Summer

Most people would agree that there are simply not enough summer meals to eat all the vine-ripened fresh tomatoes that one would like. At only 26 calories, no fat, and only 1 vegetable exchange for a medium-size tomato, they surely have established a permanent place in our diets.

When we were children, everyone grew tomatoes. Nowadays we also see pots of them growing on rooftop terraces, on windowsills, on fire escapes, and on the patio. We stick tomato plants into nearly every place in the garden that is sunny and has good drainage. Watering and watching our prize crop growing is a wonderfully relaxing and rewarding endeavor.

Not into gardening? The farmer's markets and supermarkets are full of luscious ripe tomatoes at reasonable prices most of the summer.

So what does one do with these beauties? Here are some of our favorite ideas:

- Eat them out of hand with a sprinkling of fresh herbs.
- Make tomato soup—cold gazpacho or hot bisque
- Stuff them—with almost anything: chicken or fish salad; pasta salad; rice or any other grain salad; other vegetables; a mixture of chopped leaf lettuce, arugula, and fresh mushrooms, drizzled with a little olive oil and a splash of balsamic vinegar; a mixture of nonfat ricotta cheese, chopped scallions, and chopped red bell pepper
- Slice them thickly and drizzle on some balsamic vinegar.
- Cut them into wedges and sprinkle with some shredded skim-milk mozzarella cheese and chopped basil.
- Make bruschetta—grilled slices of bread rubbed with garlic and brushed with a little olive oil, topped with chopped tomatoes and herbs.
- Make salsa.
- Make spaghetti sauce.
- Make ketchup, barbecue sauce, or tomato jam.
- Stew them with onions and celery.

And if you still have too many tomatoes, turn them into tomato sauce to freeze in plastic containers so you'll have the fresh taste of summer all winter long.

Quick Roasted Plum Tomatoes

These tasty tomatoes cook while you prepare the rest of your dinner. The herb and garlic addition makes them memorable.

olive oil cooking spray
2 medium plum or Roma tomatoes (6 ounces total)
½ teaspoon olive oil
1 clove garlic, minced
¼ teaspoon crushed dried herbes de provence *or your favorite herbs*
freshly ground pepper to taste

Preheat the oven to 425°F. Lightly coat a heavy baking sheet with cooking spray. Place the tomatoes on the sheet, drizzle with oil, and sprinkle with the garlic and herbs. Sprinkle pepper on top. Bake for 20 minutes.

Makes 2 servings.

PER SERVING: 30 calories (30% calories from fat), 1 g total fat (0.2 g saturated fat), 1 g protein, 5 g carbohydrates, 1 g dietary fiber, 0 cholesterol, 8 mg sodium

JOSLIN EXCHANGE: 1 vegetable

Roasted Zucchini with Yogurt

Once you've tried this combination, you may wish to try yogurt and herbs with different vegetables, such as asparagus, cauliflower, mushrooms, peas, and other types of squash. The recipe also works with other herbs: basil, cilantro, dill, marjoram, mint, oregano, parsley, rosemary, or tarragon.

butter-flavored cooking spray
3 medium zucchini (about 8 ounces total), cut in half lengthwise and then sliced into
*   1-inch pieces*
2 tablespoons plain nonfat yogurt
¾ teaspoon minced fresh thyme or ⅛ teaspoon crushed dried
1 clove garlic, minced, or ⅛ teaspoon garlic powder

Preheat the oven to 450°F. Lightly coat a nonstick shallow baking pan with cooking spray.

Arrange the zucchini pieces in a single layer and lightly coat them with cooking spray. Roast until crisp-tender, about 5 to 6 minutes.

Meanwhile, combine the yogurt, thyme, and garlic. Toss the roasted zucchini with the yogurt mixture and serve immediately.

Makes 2 servings.

PER SERVING: 27 calories (6% calories from fat), <1 g total fat (trace saturated fat), 2 g protein, 5 g carbohydrates, 1 g dietary fiber, trace cholesterol, 15 mg sodium

JOSLIN EXCHANGES: 1 vegetable

Green Beans with Herbs

Cooking baby vegetables quickly and then flavoring them with your favorite herbs changes them from ordinary to special. Serve them hot, at room temperature, or chilled in a salad.

8 ounces young green beans, stem ends removed
olive oil cooking spray
1 scallion (white part plus 1 inch of green), finely chopped
1 clove garlic, minced, or ⅛ teaspoon garlic powder
½ to 1 teaspoon fresh chopped tarragon, thyme, or basil, or ¼ teaspoon dried
freshly ground pepper to taste
1 teaspoon white wine vinegar

Bring a saucepan of water to a boil and add the beans. Simmer until crisp-tender, about 3 minutes. Drain well and return to the saucepan. Lightly coat the beans with cooking spray. Toss with the scallion, garlic, herbs, and pepper. Sprinkle with the vinegar and serve at once.

Makes 2 servings.

PER SERVING: 39 calories (3% calories from fat), <1 g total fat (trace saturated fat), 2 g protein, 9 g carbohydrates, 4 g dietary fiber, 0 cholesterol, 8 mg sodium

JOSLIN EXCHANGES: 2 vegetable

Green Beans with Almonds and Balsamic Vinegar

These green beans are dressed for company but are simple enough to prepare that you can enjoy them anytime. Choose beans that are crisp and vivid green so you'll know they're freshly picked. Break one; if it doesn't snap, it's not fresh. You'll need to snap off the stem end, but whether you trim the little tail at the other end is up to you.

4 ounces fresh green beans
olive oil cooking spray
1 shallot, minced, or 1 tablespoon minced red onion

1½ tablespoons balsamic vinegar
½ teaspoon sliced almonds

Bring a medium saucepan of water to a boil and add the beans. Simmer until crisp-tender, about 3 minutes. Drain, rinse under cold water, and drain again. Set aside.

Lightly coat a nonstick skillet with cooking spray. Add the shallot and sauté over low heat for 2 minutes, stirring, until the shallot is limp but not brown. Add the green beans to the skillet and heat over medium heat for 2 minutes, stirring frequently. Pour in the vinegar, and after about 30 seconds, sprinkle with the almonds. Toss to coat evenly. Serve immediately.

Makes 2 servings.

PER SERVING: 40 calories (9% calories from fat), <1 g total fat (trace saturated fat), 1 g protein, 8 g carbohydrates, 2 g dietary fiber, 0 cholesterol, 6 mg sodium

JOSLIN EXCHANGES: 1 vegetable

Balsamic Vinegar

Balsamic vinegar is an intense, sweet-tart vinegar that is a boon to anyone on a special diet. Unique to the region around Modena, Italy, balsamic vinegar is made from the unfermented juice (called mosto) of the white Trebbiano grape. Boiled down to a sweet, fruity syrup, it gets its dark color and pungent sweetness from aging in barrels made from a variety of woods, with sizes graduating over a period of years.

The finished vinegar must be at least six years old. We've attended balsamic vinegar seminars where we've tasted priceless fifty- and seventy-five-year-old balsamic vinegar, but what we buy for our kitchens is only twelve years old. Look for balsamic vinegar in your supermarket or specialty foods store.

We're passionate about balsamic vinegar and use it frequently for salads, with vegetables (it's particularly wonderful on baked onions), and sprinkled on fresh fruit—raspberries, peaches, pineapple, melon, or strawberries, with a little cracked black pepper. *Supremo* as dessert.

Summer Vegetable Stir-Fry

In the summer when friends and neighbors harvest and share their vegetables, we all benefit. Here we use the Asian method of stir-fry cooking, which allows the freshness of the ingredients to shine.

butter-flavored cooking spray
1 scallion (white part plus 1 inch of green), thinly sliced
1 medium zucchini (6 ounces), diced
1 ear of corn (3 ounces), husked and kernels removed
½ medium red bell pepper, diced
2 tablespoons shredded fresh basil
freshly ground pepper to taste

Lightly coat a large nonstick skillet or wok with the cooking spray. Place over high heat and add the scallion, zucchini, corn, and bell pepper. Stir-fry until the vegetables are crisp-cooked, 2 to 3 minutes. Remove from the heat and stir in the basil and pepper. Serve hot, warm, or cold.

Makes 2 servings.

PER SERVING: 56 calories (9% calories from fat), 1 g total fat (0.1 g saturated), 3 g protein, 12 g carbohydrates, 3 g dietary fiber, 0 cholesterol, 10 mg sodium

JOSLIN EXCHANGES: 2 vegetable

Minted Carrots and Orange

When our markets started selling bags of already-peeled baby carrots at a reasonable price, we fell in love with carrots all over again. The little finger-sized carrots are particularly sweet and have an affinity for the flavors of mint and orange without losing their individuality.

⅓ of a 16-ounce bag (about 1 cup) peeled baby carrots
butter-flavored cooking spray
1 navel orange (8 ounces), peel completely removed, sectioned
1½ tablespoons chopped fresh mint

Boil the carrots in water to cover until tender-crisp, about 4 to 5 minutes. Drain well.

Lightly coat a small nonstick sauté pan with cooking spray. Add the cooked carrots and sauté over medium heat for 1 minute. Add the orange segments and any juice you can squeeze from the membranes of the orange. Add the mint and raise the heat to high. Cook and stir until the liquid has evaporated, about 1 minute.

Makes 2 servings.

PER SERVING: 82 calories (5% calories from fat), <1 g total fat (0.1 g saturated fat), 2 g protein, 19 g carbohydrates, 4 g dietary fiber, 0 cholesterol, 29 mg sodium

JOSLIN EXCHANGES: 1 carbohydrate (1 fruit), 1 vegetable

Dinner Salads and Light Dressings

Low in calories and high in fiber, dinner salads are a godsend for anyone on a special diet. If there is time, we serve the salad before the main course, but we often eat it alongside the meal. Either way, just make sure the greens, the basis of most salads, are fresh and all the other ingredients are crisp.

There has been a revolution at the supermarket with the introduction of packaged fresh vegetables and salads. The busy shopper can buy crudités ready for the table, shredded cabbage or broccoli ready for slaw, fat-free Caesar salads in a plastic bag complete with croutons and dressing, fat-free romaine salad with raspberry vinaigrette, and mesclun, romaine hearts, broccoli florets, minced garlic, sun-dried tomatoes . . . the list goes on and on. Most of these packaged goods are more costly than if you were to purchase them in bulk; convenience costs.

Examine the complete salad packages and processed foods carefully. Both the regular and fat-free can be too high in sodium for individuals on a sodium-restricted diet. Refer to Reading Food Labels (page 20) for more information regarding the nutrient content of packaged foods.

There is a wealth of salad greens available at even the smallest supermarket. Forget ho-hum iceberg lettuce and try arugula, beet greens, Belgian endive, Boston lettuce, chard, Chinese (napa) cabbage, chicory, Bibb lettuce, escarole, kale, mesclun (a blend of eight to twelve baby lettuces, wild greens, savory herbs, and edible petals), mustard greens, pea shoots, radicchio, romaine lettuce, spinach, sprouts, and watercress.

Keep the dressing light, using no more than 1 tablespoon per cup of greens. Here are some sassy dressings that we use.

Tomato Buttermilk
In a small bowl, whisk together ⅓ cup of buttermilk, 1 tablespoon of tomato paste, 1 teaspoon of grated onion, and ½ teaspoon of dried crushed tarragon (or basil). Transfer to a jar with a tight-fitting lid to chill until ready to use.

Makes about ⅓ cup.

PER 2 TABLESPOONS: 20 calories (16% calories from fat), <1 g total fat (0.2 g saturated fat), 1 g protein, 3 g carbohydrates, 0 dietary fiber, 1 mg cholesterol, 86 mg sodium

JOSLIN EXCHANGES: free

Creamy Honey Dijon

In a small bowl, whisk together ½ cup of plain nonfat yogurt, 1 tablespoon of Dijon mustard, ½ tablespoon of balsamic vinegar, and ½ tablespoon of honey. Transfer to a jar with a tight-fitting lid to chill until ready to use.

Makes about ½ cup.

PER 2 TABLESPOONS: 32 calories (11% calories from fat), 1 g total fat (trace saturated fat), 2 g protein, 6 g carbohydrates, 0 dietary fiber, 1 mg cholesterol, 104 mg sodium

JOSLIN EXCHANGES: free

Orange Sesame Dressing

In a small bowl, whisk together ¼ cup of fresh orange juice, 2 tablespoons of sherry wine vinegar, 1 teaspoon of minced orange zest, 1 teaspoon of canola oil, ⅛ teaspoon of dark sesame oil, and ¼ teaspoon of sesame seeds. Transfer to a jar with a tight-fitting lid to chill until ready to use.

Makes about ⅓ cup.

PER 2 TABLESPOONS: 36 calories (16% calories from fat), 1 g total fat (0.2 g saturated fat), 0 protein, 2 g carbohydrates, 0 dietary fiber, 0 cholesterol, 0 sodium

JOSLIN EXCHANGES: free

Roquefort or Blue Cheese Dressing

In a small bowl, whisk together ½ cup of 1% buttermilk, 1 tablespoon of crumbled Roquefort or blue cheese, 1 teaspoon of grated onion, and freshly ground pepper to taste. Transfer to a jar with a tight-fitting lid to chill until ready to use.

Makes about ½ cup.

PER 2 TABLESPOONS: 20 calories (45% calories from fat), 1 g total fat (0.6 g saturated fat), 2 g protein, 2 g carbohydrates, 0 dietary fiber, 2 mg cholesterol, 70 mg sodium

JOSLIN EXCHANGES: free

French Vinaigrette

In a small bowl, whisk together 2 tablespoons of olive oil, 2 tablespoons of red wine vinegar, 1 tablespoon of water, 1 teaspoon of minced shallots, ¼ teaspoon of Dijon mustard, and freshly ground pepper to taste. Transfer to a jar with a tight-fitting lid to chill until ready to use.

Makes about ⅓ cup.

PER 2 TABLESPOONS: 102 calories (93% calories from fat), 10 g total fat (1.4 g saturated fat), 0 protein, 2 g carbohydrates, 0 dietary fiber, 0 cholesterol, 12 mg sodium

JOSLIN EXCHANGES: 2 fat

Lemon-Balsamic Dressing

In a food processor or blender, process 3 tablespoons of fresh lemon juice, 2 tablespoons of balsamic vinegar, 2 peeled cloves of garlic, and 1½ teaspoons of crushed dried basil until smooth. Transfer to a jar with a tight-fitting lid to chill until ready to use.

Makes about ⅓ cup.

PER 2 TABLESPOONS: 28 calories (2% calories from fat), 0 total fat (0 saturated fat), 0 protein, 6 g carbohydrates, 0 dietary fiber, 0 cholesterol, 4 mg sodium

JOSLIN EXCHANGES: free

Raspberry Vinaigrette

In a food processor or blender, process ½ cup of fresh or frozen (no-sugar-added and thawed) raspberries and 2 tablespoons of white wine vinegar for 30 seconds. Strain through a fine sieve to remove the seeds; discard the seeds. Transfer to a jar with a tight-fitting lid and whisk in 1 tablespoon of canola oil. Taste. If the raspberries are very sour, add ½ packet of sugar substitute.

Makes about ⅓ cup.

PER 2 TABLESPOONS: 64 calories (73% calories from fat), 6 g total fat (0.4 g saturated fat), 0 protein, 4 g carbohydrates, 0 dietary fiber, 0 cholesterol, 0 sodium

JOSLIN EXCHANGES: 1 fat

Cucumber, Sweet Onion, and Cherry Tomato Salad

Lovely sweet onions such as the Vidalia, Maui, Walla Walla, or Texas 1015 Super-sweet are available at your market from early spring to late fall. Try baking the leftover onion in aluminum foil, splashed with balsamic vinegar, for another meal. You'll be surprised at its mild taste.

1 large cucumber, peeled and thinly sliced
¼ large sweet onion, peeled, cut thin, and broken into rings
8 cherry tomatoes, cut in half

Dressing:

1½ teaspoons red wine vinegar
½ teaspoon canola oil
2 tablespoons plain nonfat yogurt
½ teaspoon Dijon mustard
1 clove garlic, minced, or ⅛ teaspoon garlic powder
1 teaspoon chopped fresh tarragon or ⅓ teaspoon crushed dried
freshly ground pepper to taste

4 Boston lettuce leaves, crisped

Place the cucumber, onion, and cherry tomatoes in a bowl.

In a small bowl or cup, combine the vinegar, canola oil, yogurt, mustard, garlic, tarragon, and pepper. Mix well with a fork. Pour over the vegetables and toss to coat.

Place 2 lettuce leaves on each of 2 salad plates to form a lettuce cup. Mound the salad in each cup.

Makes 2 servings.

PER SERVING: 71 calories (20% calories from fat), 2 g total fat (0.2 g saturated fat), 3 g protein, 13 g carbohydrates, 3 g dietary fiber, trace cholesterol, 30 mg sodium

JOSLIN EXCHANGES: 2 vegetable

Carrot and Apple Salad

Refreshing bits of apple add the right touch to this simple salad. Serve the salad as an accompaniment for grilled chicken or pork.

1 large carrot, pared and coarsely grated
1 small unpeeled Granny Smith apple, cored and finely chopped

Dressing:

2½ teaspoons fresh lemon juice
½ teaspoon ground cinnamon
1½ tablespoons shredded fresh mint

Place the carrot and apple in a small bowl. In a cup, combine the lemon juice, cinnamon, and mint. Pour over the carrot and apples and stir to coat evenly. Serve at once.

Makes 2 servings.

PER SERVING: 70 calories (5% calories from fat), <1 g total fat (trace saturated fat), <1 g protein, 17 g carbohydrates, 4 g dietary fiber, 0 cholesterol, 21 mg sodium

JOSLIN EXCHANGES: 1 carbohydrate (1 fruit)

Fruit Salads by the Season

Winter

Segment ½ of a medium grapefruit, ½ of a medium navel orange. Slice 1 small banana. Arrange the fruit in a single layer in a shallow baking dish. Sprinkle with cinnamon and drizzle with 1 teaspoon of honey. Broil until the fruit is lightly brown. Serve warm in small bowls.

Makes 2 servings.

PER SERVING: 74 calories (3% calories from fat), <1 g total fat (trace saturated fat), 1 g protein, 19 g carbohydrates, 2 g dietary fiber, 0 cholesterol, 1 mg sodium

JOSLIN EXCHANGES: 1 carbohydrate (1 fruit)

Spring

In a medium bowl, combine 1 cup of sliced strawberries, ½ cup of diced mango, and ¼ teaspoon of grated lemon zest. Just before serving sprinkle with 1 teaspoon of balsamic vinegar.

Makes 2 servings.

PER SERVING: 55 calories (6% calories from fat), <1 g total fat (0 g saturated fat), 1 g protein, 14 g carbohydrates, 2 g dietary fiber, 0 cholesterol, 2 mg sodium

JOSLIN EXCHANGES: 1 carbohydrate (1 fruit)

Summer

In a medium bowl, combine ½ cup of cold watermelon balls, ½ cup of cold cantaloupe balls, and ½ cup of cold honeydew melon balls. Sprinkle with 2 tablespoons of crumbled feta cheese and 2 tablespoons of minced fresh mint, and stir gently. Serve at once; if the salad sits, it will become watery.

Makes 2 servings.

PER SERVING: 62 calories (25% calories from fat), 2 g total fat (1.3 g saturated fat), 2 g protein, 10 g carbohydrates, 1 g dietary fiber, 6 mg cholesterol, 86 mg sodium

JOSLIN EXCHANGE: 1 carbohydrate (1 fruit)

Fall

Quarter and core a large red apple; do not peel. Cut each quarter into ¼-inch slices. Place in a small bowl and mix with 1 tablespoon of lemon juice. Arrange 2 washed and crisped Boston lettuce leaves on each of 2 salad plates. Top with apple slices, fanning them out to form an attractive pattern. In a small bowl, whisk together 1 tablespoon of canola oil, 1 tablespoon of balsamic vinegar, and 1 teaspoon of Dijon mustard. Drizzle the mixture over the apples and serve. Sprinkle with freshly ground pepper to taste.

Makes 2 servings.

PER SERVING: 116 calories (56% calories from fat), 7 g total fat (0.5 g saturated fat), 0 protein, 13 g carbohydrates, 1 g dietary fiber, 0 cholesterol, 65 mg sodium

JOSLIN EXCHANGES: 1 carbohydrate (1 fruit), 1 fat

Beet and Orange Salad

Served as a separate first course, this is an elegant salad. When time is short, everything can be tossed together in a salad bowl and eaten alongside the main course.

> *2 cups baby mixed greens*
> *1 medium navel orange*
> *2 ounces canned sliced beets*
> *2 tablespoons minced red onion*
> *½ tablespoon fresh orange juice*
> *½ teaspoon fresh lemon juice*
> *1½ tablespoons olive oil*
> *salt (optional)*
> *freshly ground pepper to taste*
> *1 teaspoon minced fresh parsley for garnish (optional)*

Lightly rinse salad greens. Wrap in paper towels and refrigerate until ready to serve.

Working over a bowl so you can catch the juice, cut the peel from the orange with a sharp knife, making sure you remove all of the white pith. Slice the orange crosswise into ¼-inch rounds and arrange on 1 side of each of 2 large salad plates alternating with slices of beet. Sprinkle with the red onion. Cover loosely with plastic wrap and refrigerate for at least 10 minutes and up to 1 hour.

To make the dressing, whisk together the orange juice, lemon juice, and olive oil in a small bowl. Season with salt (if using) and pepper.

To serve, arrange the salad greens on the side of the orange-beet slices. Drizzle dressing over all and sprinkle with parsley if desired. Serve immediately.

Makes 2 servings.

PER SERVING: 145 calories (61% calories from fat), 10 g total fat (1.4 g saturated fat), 2 g protein, 13 g carbohydrates, 3 g dietary fiber, 0 cholesterol, 92 mg sodium

JOSLIN EXCHANGES: ½ carbohydrate (½ fruit), 1 vegetable, 2 fat

Chopped Salad with Low-Fat Ranch Dressing

This is a colorful salad to serve with plain meat, fish, or fowl. This dressing is also delicious on a bed of fresh spinach with sliced mushrooms.

Chopped salad:

1 cup chopped romaine and radicchio
½ small red bell pepper, seeded and coarsely chopped
½ small yellow bell pepper, seeded and coarsely chopped
½ small green bell pepper, seeded and coarsely chopped
4 radishes, trimmed and thinly sliced
¼ cup mung bean sprouts

Low-fat ranch dressing:

3 tablespoons 1% buttermilk
1 tablespoon reduced-calorie mayonnaise
1 teaspoon white wine vinegar
1 scallion (white part only), minced
dash garlic powder
dash onion powder

1 hard-cooked egg white, chopped

In a medium salad bowl, combine all the ingredients for the salad except the egg white. Toss. In a small bowl, whisk together the dressing ingredients.

To serve, divide the salad between 2 salad plates. Spoon on the dressing and top with some of the hard-cooked egg white.

Makes 2 servings.

PER SERVING: 64 calories (26% calories from fat), 2 g total fat (0.4 g saturated fat), 4 g protein, 8 g carbohydrates, 2 g dietary fiber, 3 mg cholesterol, 122 mg sodium

JOSLIN EXCHANGES: ½ very low fat protein, 1 vegetable

2 TABLESPOONS DRESSING: 29 calories (52% calories from fat), 2 g total fat (0.4 g saturated fat), 1 g protein, 3 g carbohydrates, 0 dietary fiber, 3 mg cholesterol, 63 mg sodium

JOSLIN EXCHANGES: free

Jicama Slaw

Dean Fearing serves a similar salad from his kitchen at The Mansion on Turtle Creek in Dallas, Texas. It's a fiesta of color and fresh taste.

½ cup peeled and shredded jicama
½ cup peeled and shredded carrot
½ cup unpeeled and shredded zucchini
½ small red bell pepper, seeded and cut into fine julienne strips
1 tablespoon minced fresh cilantro
1 teaspoon canola oil
1½ teaspoons fresh lime juice
dash cayenne pepper

In a medium bowl, combine all the ingredients. Toss to mix well. Serve at once.

Makes 2 servings.

PER SERVING: 54 calories (38% calories from fat), 2 g total fat (0.2 g saturated fat), 1 g protein, 8 g carbohydrates, 3 g dietary fiber, 0 cholesterol, 12 mg sodium

JOSLIN EXCHANGES: 1 vegetable

Snow Pea Salad

We toss blanched snow peas with other crisp vegetables for a delicious salad. Fresh cilantro gives it a distinct taste, but if it's too strong for you or unavailable, try adding fresh mint.

3 ounces fresh snow pea pods, strings removed
3 ounces fresh bean sprouts
1 scallion (white part plus 1 inch of green), thinly sliced
½ tablespoon finely chopped fresh cilantro, or to taste

Dressing:

½ teaspoon low-sodium soy sauce
¼ teaspoon powdered ginger
1 tablespoon rice vinegar or cider vinegar
4 drops sesame oil
1 teaspoon canola oil
1 tablespoon water
freshly ground pepper to taste

2 lettuce cups
1 teaspoon sesame seeds, toasted

Place the snow peas in a colander and pour boiling water over to blanch them. Refresh under cold water or toss with ice cubes. Place the snow peas on a towel to dry.

In a serving bowl, combine the snow peas, bean sprouts, scallion, and cilantro.

Whisk together the dressing ingredients in a small bowl. Pour over the vegetables and toss to coat evenly. Divide the vegetables evenly between the lettuce cups. Sprinkle with sesame seeds and serve. (This salad will keep in the refrigerator for 2 hours if necessary.)

Makes 2 servings.

PER SERVING: 71 calories (42% calories from fat), 3 g total fat (0.3 g saturated fat), 4 g protein, 8 g carbohydrates, 3 g dietary fiber, 0 cholesterol, 52 mg sodium

JOSLIN EXCHANGES: 2 vegetable

Summer Salad

This incredibly good salad relies on the freshest tomatoes and basil you can find. Make it often while the ingredients are at their best. ¶ If you're too tired or it's too hot to cook, you can turn this salad into a whole meal by adding a well-drained 6-ounce can of water-packed tuna when you add the croutons. That will add per serving 98 calories, 1 gram of fat, 22 grams of protein, and 3 very low fat protein exchanges.

Shallot dressing:

½ tablespoon minced shallot
¼ teaspoon minced garlic
1 tablespoon olive oil
1 tablespoon balsamic vinegar
⅛ teaspoon salt (optional)
freshly ground pepper to taste

Salad:

1 large firm, ripe tomato, coarsely chopped
1 small red onion, coarsely chopped
1 small cucumber, peeled, seeded, and coarsely chopped
1 small red bell pepper, seeded and coarsely chopped
6 large fresh basil leaves, shredded
1 cup fat-free croutons
4 pitted black ripe olives, quartered (optional)

In a small bowl, whisk together the dressing ingredients. Set aside to allow the flavors to blend while you make the salad.

In a medium salad bowl, combine the tomato, onion, cucumber, bell pepper, and basil. Drizzle with the dressing and toss to coat evenly. Add the croutons and olives (if using). Toss again. Let the salad sit at room temperature for at least 15 minutes before serving. Toss again just before serving.

Makes 2 servings.

PER SERVING: 191 calories (38% calories from fat), 7 g total fat (1.3 g saturated fat), 4 g protein, 27 g carbohydrates, 4 g dietary fiber, 0 cholesterol, 119 mg sodium

JOSLIN EXCHANGES: 1 carbohydrate (1 bread/starch), 2 vegetable, 1 fat

1½ TABLESPOONS DRESSING: 72 calories (84% calories from fat), 7 g total fat (0.9 g saturated fat), 0 protein, 3 g carbohydrates, 0 dietary fiber, 0 cholesterol, 2 mg sodium

JOSLIN EXCHANGES: 1 fat

Broccoli and Red Pepper Salad

The benefit of broccoli in the diet as an antioxidant is well known. The problem is varying the way we serve it. Here we have a Mediterranean salad served at room temperature that is also excellent chilled. The olives are available in bulk at many grocery store delis.

6 ounces broccoli florets with 1-inch stem
½ red bell pepper, cored, seeded, membranes removed, and sliced in ¼-inch julienne strips
1 tablespoon olive oil
1 tablespoon red wine vinegar
2 cloves garlic, minced, or ¼ teaspoon garlic powder
⅛ teaspoon kosher salt (optional)
freshly ground pepper to taste
½ tablespoon chopped Greek or Italian black olives

Place the broccoli florets in a covered microwave-safe dish. Place 1 tablespoon of water in the dish, cover, and cook in the microwave on HIGH for 1 minute. Test to see the degree of doneness. Stir the broccoli and cook 45 seconds more, until cooked but still crisp to the bite. Refresh the broccoli with cold water, drain, and place on a serving plate. Place the bell pepper strips on the broccoli.

Combine the oil, vinegar, garlic, salt (if using), and pepper to make a vinaigrette. Drizzle over the vegetables and garnish with the chopped olives. Serve warm or chill for later use.

Makes 2 servings.

PER SERVING: 112 calories (56% calories from fat), 8 g total fat (1.0 g saturated fat), 3 g protein, 10 g carbohydrates, 3 g dietary fiber, 0 cholesterol, 59 mg sodium

JOSLIN EXCHANGES: 2 vegetable, 1 fat

Mediterranean Salad

This is a refreshingly different salad. Another time, prepare a double recipe of the dressing to use as a marinade for grilling chicken, shrimp, or vegetables.

1 medium tomato, seeded and chopped
1 scallion (white part plus 1 inch of green), chopped
½ cucumber, peeled, seeded, and sliced paper-thin
2 tablespoons minced green bell pepper

Dressing:

1½ tablespoons plain nonfat yogurt
2¼ teaspoons lemon juice
⅛ teaspoon minced garlic
¼ teaspoon ground cumin
1 teaspoon fresh mint, shredded, plus extra for garnish
⅛ teaspoon salt (optional)
freshly ground pepper to taste

In a medium bowl, combine the tomato, scallion, cucumber, and bell pepper.

In a small bowl, mix together the yogurt, lemon juice, garlic, cumin, mint, salt (if using), and pepper. Toss with the vegetables and serve.

Makes 2 servings.

PER SERVING: 44 calories (10% calories from fat), <1 g total fat (0.1 g saturated fat), 2 g protein, 9 g carbohydrates, 2 g dietary fiber, 0 cholesterol, 22 mg sodium

JOSLIN EXCHANGES: 2 vegetable

DESSERTS

Blackberry Cobbler

This is a delightful cobbler that can also be made with fresh blueberries, raspberries, sliced fresh peaches, or sliced fresh plums. It's quite rich, so a small portion is plenty. ❡ The cobbler serves six, so plan to make it when you have company, or you will have leftovers.

vegetable cooking spray
1 cup fresh blackberries
2 teaspoons grated orange zest
2 tablespoons sugar
2 tablespoons canola oil
1 large egg
½ cup unbleached all-purpose flour
¾ teaspoon baking powder
⅛ teaspoon salt
¼ cup evaporated skim milk

Preheat the oven to 350° Lightly coat a 6-inch round metal baking pan with cooking spray. Spread the blackberries in the pan and sprinkle with 1 teaspoon of the grated zest.

In a medium bowl, cream together the sugar and oil. Whisk in the egg until the mixture is thick and smooth. Sift together the flour, baking powder, and salt. Add to the egg mixture, alternating with the milk, until well combined. Stir in the remaining 1 teaspoon of grated zest.

Spread the mixture over the blackberries. Bake for 20 to 25 minutes, until a tester inserted in the middle comes out clean. Cool in the pan on a wire rack before serving. To serve, spoon into small dessert bowls.

Makes 6 servings.

PER SERVING: 128 calories (42% calories from fat), 6 g total fat (0.6 g saturated fat), 3 g protein, 17 g carbohydrates, 1 g dietary fiber, 108 mg cholesterol, 127 mg sodium

JOSLIN EXCHANGES: 1 carbohydrate (1 bread/starch), 1 fat

Individual Cheesecakes

With the growing availability of fat-free and lower-fat products in the grocery store, you can enjoy cheesecake that is good tasting without feeling deprived of dessert.

1 teaspoon graham cracker crumbs
2 ounces fat-free cream cheese
½ ounce reduced-fat cream cheese
1 tablespoon fat-free sour cream
2 teaspoons sugar
2 teaspoons grated orange rind
2 tablespoons egg substitute
¼ cup fresh berries such as blueberries or raspberries

Place 2 paper baking cup liners (2½-inch size) in 2 microwave-safe baking cups. Divide the graham cracker crumbs between the 2 cups and set aside.

Place all the ingredients except the berries in a medium bowl. Beat with an electric mixer until fluffy and well blended, about 2 minutes. Spoon the mixture into the paper cup liners, filling the cups ⅔ full.

Place in the microwave and cook at MEDIUM for 90 seconds. Turn the cups and continue to cook at MEDIUM for 1 minute, or until the top is firm.

Remove from the oven and cool on a rack. When ready to serve, remove the cheesecakes from the baking cups. Serve with berries alongside.

Makes 2 servings.

PER SERVING: 90 calories (17% calories from fat), 2 g total fat (0.5 g saturated fat), 7 g protein, 11 g carbohydrates, 1 g dietary fiber, 2 mg cholesterol, 230 mg sodium

JOSLIN EXCHANGES: ½ very low fat protein, 1 carbohydrate (1 bread/starch)

Pineapple Upside-Down Cake

This is a lightened version of an old-fashioned favorite. The cake adequately serves three; ask a neighbor or friend to stop by for dessert so you're not tempted to keep nibbling.

butter-flavored cooking spray
1 teaspoon reduced-calorie margarine
1 teaspoon dark brown sugar
½ cup crushed pineapple packed in natural juice, drained
½ cup unbleached all-purpose flour
2 tablespoons sugar
½ teaspoon baking powder
1 egg, slightly beaten
1 tablespoon canola oil
½ teaspoon vanilla extract
⅓ cup evaporated skim milk

Preheat the oven to 350°F. Lightly coat a 2-cup baking dish with cooking spray.

Combine the margarine and brown sugar. Spread evenly over the bottom of the prepared baking dish. Top with the pineapple.

Sift together the flour, sugar, and baking powder in a medium mixing bowl. In a separate bowl, combine the egg, canola oil, vanilla extract, and evaporated milk. Stir into the dry ingredients, beating until smooth. Pour the batter over the pineapple. Bake for 25 to 30 minutes, until a tester inserted in the center comes out clean.

Remove from the oven and immediately invert onto a serving plate. Leave the baking dish on the cake to allow the sugar and pineapple mixtures to drain onto the top of the cake as it cools. Cool for at least 15 minutes before removing the dish. Serve warm or at room temperature.

Makes 3 servings.

PER SERVING: 191 calories (13% calories from fat), 3 g total fat (0.8 g saturated fat), 6 g protein, 35 g carbohydrates, 1 g dietary fiber, 72 mg cholesterol, 153 mg sodium

JOSLIN EXCHANGES: 2½ carbohydrate (2 bread/starch, ½ fruit)

Apple Tarts

Some desserts lose their fabulous flavor and visual appeal when modified for a diabetic diet, but here's one that looks and tastes just as you remembered.

1 sheet frozen puff pastry dough
1 6-ounce tart apple such as Gala or Granny Smith
1 teaspoon grated lemon zest
½ teaspoon fresh lemon juice
butter-flavored cooking spray
2 tablespoons unsweetened applesauce
1 teaspoon sugar
⅛ teaspoon nutmeg

Open the sealed puff pastry package. It will be folded in thirds. With a sharp-pointed knife, cut along 1 fold to separate ⅓ of the dough. Cut that third into 2 equal pieces. Seal and refreeze the remaining dough.

Preheat the oven to 450°F.

While the oven is heating, pare, quarter, core, and thinly slice the apple. Sprinkle the lemon zest and lemon juice on the apple.

When the oven is hot, lightly roll the dough pieces to form two 4½-inch squares. Place the dough pieces on a nonstick cookie sheet that has been coated with cooking spray. Lightly coat the dough with cooking spray. Top each half of the dough with the applesauce, sugar, nutmeg, and apple slices, leaving a ½-inch border. Coat once again with cooking spray.

Bake for 15 minutes. Check after 10 minutes and lower the heat to 425°F. Bake until the crust is golden and some of the apple edges have browned. Serve warm.

Makes 2 servings.

PER SERVING: 178 calories (30% calories from fat), 6 g total fat (1.3 g saturated fat), 2 g protein, 29 g carbohydrates, 4 g dietary fiber, 0 cholesterol, 68 mg sodium

JOSLIN EXCHANGES: 2 carbohydrate (1 bread/starch, 1 fruit), 1 fat

Individual Ice Cream Bombes

These easy-to-make ice cream desserts make an elegant ending to any meal. Use contrasting colored ice cream (your choice of flavors) for the best effect. We use cherry and chocolate flavors in this recipe, but you can certainly add a third flavor, such as vanilla, for more taste. Just make sure the total amount is no more than 6 ounces. ❡ To facilitate freezing and easy removal from the mold, use an ice cream with no fruits or nuts for the outer layer. You'll need two 6-ounce freezer-proof molds or soufflé cups to make this recipe.

vegetable cooking spray
4 strips waxed paper, 2 inches by 12 inches wide
3 ounces chocolate-flavored fat-free, no-sugar-added ice cream
3 ounces cherry-flavored fat-free, no-sugar-added ice cream

Lightly coat the molds with cooking spray. Place 2 waxed paper strips in an ✕ in each mold with the ends hanging over the top.

Spoon the chocolate or first flavor of ice cream into the molds, forming a layer on the bottom and sides, and making sure not to leave air bubbles. Place in the freezer to harden for 3 to 5 minutes. Remove from the freezer and fill the molds with the cherry or second flavor ice cream. (If using vanilla or a third flavor, repeat this process.) Return the molds to the freezer until ready to serve.

To unmold, invert on chilled dessert plates after running a sharp knife around the edge of the mold. Cover the mold with a kitchen towel that has been placed in hot water and then wrung out. Tap the waxed paper and the top of mold to help loosen if necessary. Remove the waxed paper strips. Serve immediately or refreeze until ready to serve.

Makes 2 servings.

PER SERVING: 108 calories (no calories from fat), 0 total fat (0 saturated fat), 4 g protein, 23 g carbohydrates, 0 dietary fiber, 0 cholesterol, 57 mg sodium

JOSLIN EXCHANGES: 1½ carbohydrate (1½ bread/starch)

Frozen Gelatin Mousse

This dessert brings back memories of the '50s. Its old-fashioned simplicity and the use of sugar-free fruit-flavored gelatin (a free food) create a dessert that you'll want to make again and again, modifying the recipe by switching flavors of ice cream and gelatin. The recipe makes enough mousse for four servings; if you're using only two, keep the remaining mousse frozen for another time. It'll keep for up to three weeks.

1 3-ounce package sugar-free strawberry-flavored gelatin
¾ cup boiling water
¾ cup ice cubes
¾ cup fat-free, no-sugar-added vanilla ice cream
2 to 4 perfect strawberries with stems

Place the gelatin in the bowl of an electric mixer and add the boiling water. Stir for 2 minutes, until the gelatin is completely dissolved. Add the ice cubes and stir until the gelatin starts to set. Remove any small pieces of ice that do not melt.

Using an electric mixer, slowly beat the gelatin and begin adding the ice cream, 1 tablespoon at a time. When all the ice cream has been added, beat the mixture for another 30 seconds. Place in the freezer for up to 1 hour.

Divide into 4 dessert glasses or dishes. Top each serving with a strawberry. Serve at once.

Makes 4 servings.

PER SERVING: 52 calories (2% calories from fat), <1 g total fat (0.1 g saturated fat), 3 g protein, 10 g carbohydrates, <1 g dietary fiber, 0 cholesterol, 73 mg sodium

JOSLIN EXCHANGES: 1 carbohydrate (1 bread/starch)

Ice Cream Sandwiches

Ice cream sandwiches can be as simple or as fancy as you wish to make them. For fancy desserts try making an open-faced sandwich, using a small scoop (melon baller) to place two or three different fat-free flavors of ice cream onto a store-bought chocolate dietetic cookie. Also try sugar-free sorbets, which are beautiful and are the delicious essence of the fruit. Top with a fresh berry and the second cookie, cut in half, placed on top like butterfly wings.

To make an old-fashioned ice cream sandwich, place ½ cup of fat-free ice cream between two of your favorite low-sugar or no-sugar cookies. Be careful to count the carbohydrates (check the Joslin Exchanges, page 249) and eat the ice cream sandwich as part of your meal. It may not be the richest dessert you have ever eaten, but it will bring back memories of hot summer evenings, no shoes, and a game of tag in the backyard.

Quick Strawberry Jubilee

This elegant topping for vanilla ice cream is traditionally made with pitted sweet cherries. Here we substitute strawberries because they're available year-round both fresh and frozen. Feel free to use fresh cherries when available.

> *1 tablespoon fresh lemon juice*
> *1 tablespoon water*
> *1½ tablespoons kirsch or brandy*
> *1 cup fresh strawberries, cut in half, or frozen no-sugar-added berries*
> *1 teaspoon sugar*
> *2 ½-cup scoops nonfat sugar-free vanilla ice cream or frozen yogurt*

Heat the lemon juice, water, and 1 tablespoon of kirsch in a small skillet. Add the strawberries, raise the heat, and boil until most of the liquid evaporates. Sprinkle with the sugar and add the remaining ½ tablespoon of kirsch. Heat for 30 seconds. Place a scoop of ice cream or yogurt into 2 serving dishes. Ladle the strawberries and sauce over each portion.

Makes 2 servings.

PER SERVING: 146 calories (2% calories from fat), <1 g total fat (trace saturated fat), 4 g protein, 27 g carbohydrates, 1 g dietary fiber, 0 cholesterol, 51 mg sodium

JOSLIN EXCHANGES: 2 carbohydrate (1 bread/starch, 1 fruit)

Fresh Fruit Crisps

This versatile dessert can be modified to use fresh fruit for any season of the year. Try your favorite apples or peaches with fresh or frozen raspberries, or strawberries or apricots with blueberries.

butter-flavored cooking spray
1 4-ounce Bartlett pear, peeled, quartered, pared, and cut in 1-inch pieces
½ cup fresh blackberries
1 tablespoon fresh lemon juice
½ teaspoon grated lemon zest

Streusel topping:

1 packet sugar substitute
½ teaspoon sugar
½ teaspoon ground cinnamon
⅛ teaspoon ground nutmeg
1½ tablespoons all-purpose flour
1 tablespoon rolled oats
1 tablespoon reduced-fat margarine

Preheat the oven to 425° F. Coat 2 ⅔-cup soufflé dishes or ovenproof dessert cups with cooking spray.

Combine the fruit with the lemon juice and rind. Divide evenly between the 2 dessert cups.

Using a fork or your fingers, combine the sugar substitute, sugar, cinnamon, nutmeg, flour, oats, and margarine to make a crumble topping. Sprinkle on top of the fruit. Bake until crisp and the fruit is cooked, about 15 minutes. Cool on a wire rack. Serve warm.

Makes 2 servings.

PER SERVING: 119 calories (24% calories from fat), 3 g total fat (0.5 g saturated fat), 2 g protein, 22 g carbohydrates, 4 g dietary fiber, 0 cholesterol, 68 mg sodium

JOSLIN EXCHANGES: 1½ carbohydrate (½ bread/starch, 1 fruit)

Frozen Grapes

Frozen grapes are a particularly welcome dessert on a hot summer evening, but they also make a superb ending to a spicy meal at other times of the year.

Just pick the seedless grapes off the stem and place them on a rimmed baking sheet lined with paper towels. Freeze until hard; it takes about an hour. Once frozen, transfer the grapes to a self-sealing plastic freezer bag.

When ready to serve, pile the frozen grapes into pretty dessert goblets or dishes. We like to mix the colors—red, green, and black. Just remember, fifteen grapes are about 60 calories and 15 grams of carbohydrate, making 1 carbohydrate (1 fruit) exchange.

Quick Rice Pudding

This is a creamy rice pudding that takes only minutes to make.

1 cup evaporated skim milk
¼ cup cooked white rice
½ of a 1-ounce package sugar-free vanilla pudding mix
2 tablespoons golden raisins
nutmeg for sprinkling

Combine all the ingredients except the nutmeg in a 1-quart glass measuring cup or microwave-safe bowl. Cover with a sheet of waxed paper and microwave on MEDIUM for 11 to 13 minutes, stirring 3 times, until the pudding is thickened. Let stand at room temperature for 5 minutes. Serve warm or chilled, sprinkled with nutmeg.

Makes 3 servings.

PER SERVING: 124 calories (2% calories from fat), <1 g total fat (0.1 g saturated fat), 7 g protein, 24 g carbohydrates, <1 g dietary fiber, 3 mg cholesterol, 293 mg sodium

JOSLIN EXCHANGES: 1½ carbohydrate (½ nonfat milk, 1 bread/starch)

Tapioca Pudding with Berries

For most of us, tapioca pudding is old-fashioned comfort food. When you sprinkle fresh berries of the season on top, it makes it special.

2 tablespoons quick-cooking tapioca
2 teaspoons sugar
1 packet sugar substitute
1 large egg
1 cup skim milk
½ teaspoon vanilla extract
⅓ cup fresh berries (blackberries, raspberries, blueberries, or sliced strawberries),
*   rinsed*

Combine the tapioca, sugar, sugar substitute, egg, and milk in a medium microwave-safe bowl. Whisk until smooth. Microwave on HIGH, uncovered, for 8 minutes. Whisk until smooth. Microwave on HIGH for another 2 to 3 minutes, until the mixture is boiling. Remove from the microwave and stir in the vanilla extract. Pour the mixture into 2 dessert dishes, cover with plastic wrap, and refrigerate for at least 20 minutes. Just before serving, sprinkle each dish with half of the berries.

Makes 2 servings.

PER SERVING: 152 calories (17% calories from fat), 3 g total fat (0.9 g saturated fat), 8 g protein, 24 g carbohydrates, 1 g dietary fiber, 108 mg cholesterol, 96 mg sodium

JOSLIN EXCHANGES: 1½ carbohydrate (½ nonfat milk, 1 bread/starch)

Old-Fashioned Bread Pudding

Crisp on the top and creamy inside, this old-fashioned treat is a welcome dessert anytime of year. You can make it with dried cherries, as we've done here, or raisins, dried blueberries, or chopped dried apricots.

butter-flavored cooking spray
1 cup cubed day-old French bread (toasted if bread is fresh)
1 cup skim milk
½ teaspoon reduced-calorie margarine
½ teaspoon grated orange zest
½ tablespoon chopped dried cherries (no sugar added)
⅛ teaspoon vanilla extract
½ teaspoon ground cinnamon
½ teaspoon sugar substitute, or to taste
2 tablespoons egg substitute

Preheat the oven to 375°F. Lightly coat 2 2-cup soufflé dishes with cooking spray.

Divide the bread cubes between the prepared dishes. In a small saucepan, combine the milk and margarine. Scald the milk. Remove from the heat and stir in the orange zest, cherries, vanilla extract, cinnamon, sugar substitute, and egg substitute. Pour over the bread cubes.

Place the soufflé dishes on a baking sheet since the mixture may bubble over. Bake for 20 minutes, until the top is crisp and a knife inserted in the center comes out clean. Serve warm.

Makes 2 servings.

PER SERVING: 147 calories (13% calories from fat), 2 g total fat (0.6 g saturated fat), 9 g protein, 23 g carbohydrates, 1 g dietary fiber, 2 mg cholesterol, 274 mg sodium

JOSLIN EXCHANGES: 1½ carbohydrate (½ nonfat milk, 1 bread/starch)

Sautéed Banana with Crème Fraîche

We keep tangy low-fat crème fraîche in the refrigerator to use with fresh fruits, to add to flavored vinegar for a salad dressing, and to top vegetables and soups. Our recipe for crème fraîche, which follows, will keep in the refrigerator for at least a week.

butter-flavored cooking spray
1 large ripe banana (5 ounces), peeled and sliced into ¼-inch slices
⅛ teaspoon ground cinnamon
2 teaspoons cognac or dark rum
½ cup Crème Fraîche (recipe follows)

Coat a nonstick sauté pan with cooking spray. Add the banana and sauté over medium-high heat for 1 minute. Sprinkle with cinnamon and cognac. Raise the heat and sauté until evaporated. Arrange the banana slices in 2 dessert dishes and top with the crème fraîche.

Makes 2 servings.

PER SERVING: 100 calories (11% calories from fat), 1 g total fat (0.7 g saturated fat), 4 g protein, 21 g carbohydrates, 2 g dietary fiber, 4 mg cholesterol, 43 mg sodium

JOSLIN EXCHANGES: 1½ carbohydrate (1 fruit, ½ nonfat milk)

Crème Fraîche

2 tablespoons 1% cultured buttermilk
2 cups plain low-fat yogurt

In a heavy saucepan, combine the buttermilk and yogurt. Heat until just lukewarm (do not overheat). Remove from the heat, cover, and let stand at room temperature for 24 hours. Refrigerate until needed.

Makes about 2 cups.

PER ¼-CUP SERVING: 35 calories (25% calories from fat), 1 g total fat (trace saturated fat), 3 g protein, 4 g carbohydrates, 0 dietary fiber, 4 mg cholesterol, 42 mg sodium

JOSLIN EXCHANGES: ½ carboyhdrate (½ nonfat milk)

Fresh Fruit for Dessert

Fresh fruit is our favorite and most frequent dessert. But instead of just eating an apple or pear, we frequently combine fruits for contrasting colors and flavors. Here are some of our favorite combinations. Each combination makes 2 servings, and each serving equals 1 carbohydrate (1 fruit) exchange.

- 1 kiwi, peeled and sliced, topped with 1 cup of fresh raspberries
- ½ cup of sliced fresh mango and ¾ cup of diced fresh pineapple, drizzled with a bit of fresh lemon juice
- 1 cup of diced, seedless watermelon and ¾ cup of fresh blackberries
- 1 carambola (star fruit), sliced, and 12 Bing cherries
- 1 small banana, sliced and sprinkled with ⅓ cup of pomegranate seeds
- 1 medium firm, ripe nectarine, sliced and topped with ¾ cup of fresh blueberries

Red, White, and Blue Parfaits

Try this dessert with a combination of your favorite fresh or frozen berries, as well as soft fruits such as peaches and melon. Rather bland frozen vanilla yogurt will sing with the flavors you add. Serve in parfait glasses or tall goblets for the prettiest effect. As a whimsy, add a small paper flag to each serving.

1½ cups fat-free, no-sugar-added frozen vanilla yogurt
⅓ cup fresh raspberries or no-sugar-added frozen
⅓ cup fresh blueberries or no-sugar-added frozen
2 perfect raspberries or blueberries for decoration

Remove the yogurt from the freezer and let stand for a few minutes to soften slightly. Divide the yogurt equally among 3 bowls. Add the raspberries to the yogurt in one bowl and mash to combine. Add the blueberries to the second bowl and mash to combine. Leave the third bowl of yogurt plain.

Quickly layer the 3 colors of yogurt in the parfait glasses starting with the raspberry (red), then the plain (white), and topping with the blueberry (blue). Decorate with perfect fruit and the paper flags. Serve at once. (If you make these before dinner, place the layered parfaits in the freezer to keep frozen. Decorate just before serving.)

Makes 2 servings.

PER SERVING: 159 calories (1% calories from fat), trace total fat (trace saturated fat), 5 g protein, 34 g carbohydrates, 2 g dietary fiber, 0 cholesterol, 76 mg sodium

JOSLIN EXCHANGES: 2 carbohydrate (1½ bread/starch, ½ fruit)

Baked Spiced Pears

Place these spiced pears in the oven just before sitting down to dinner. They'll be done when you're ready for dessert. The dessert looks fancy, but it's easy to make. Remember this recipe the next time you have company.

butter-flavored baking spray
1 firm, ripe Bartlett pear, peeled
2 teaspoons light brown sugar
½ teaspoon ground cinnamon
⅛ teaspoon ground nutmeg
1 teaspoon reduced-calorie margarine
2 ¼-cup scoops fat-free sugar-free frozen vanilla yogurt

Preheat the oven to 350°F. Lightly coat a small baking dish that is slightly larger than the pear halves laid side by side.

Halve the pear lengthwise and remove the core. Place the pears, cut side down, on a board and cut each half crosswise into 5 or 6 even slices. Take care not to cut all the way through but retain the shape of the pear half.

Using a wide spatula, transfer the pear halves to the baking dish. Mix together the brown sugar, cinnamon, and nutmeg. Sprinkle over the pears and dot each pear with half of the margarine. Bake until tender, about 20 to 25 minutes.

Remove the pears from the oven and transfer to 2 dessert plates. Serve with a scoop of the yogurt alongside.

Makes 2 servings.

PER SERVING: 118 calories (11% calories from fat), 2 g total fat (0.3 g saturated fat), 2 g protein, 26 g carbohydrates, 2 g dietary fiber, 0 cholesterol, 48 mg sodium

JOSLIN EXCHANGES: 2 carbohydrate (1 bread/starch, 1 fruit)

Roasted Pineapple, Margarita Style

No need to peel the pineapple before cooking; in fact, the peel adds to its visual appeal. This is a lovely, light way to end a meal. Put the pineapple into the oven as you're starting to eat the first course; it'll be ready when you are.

2 slices fresh ripe pineapple (about 6 ounces total), cut about 1 inch thick
2 teaspoons gold tequila
salt to taste (optional)
1 teaspoon light brown sugar
1 tablespoon fresh lime juice

Preheat the oven to 500°F. Place a single sheet of heavy-duty aluminum foil on a baking sheet.

Rub the pineapple slices with the tequila. Sprinkle with salt (if using) and place in a single layer on the prepared baking sheet. Roast, uncovered, for 15 minutes. Turn the slices over and continue to roast for another 10 minutes.

Remove from the oven and sprinkle with brown sugar and lime juice. Serve at once.

Makes 2 servings.

PER SERVING: 60 calories (6% calories from fat), <1 g total fat (trace saturated fat), 0 protein, 13 g carbohydrates, 1 g dietary fiber, 0 cholesterol, 2 mg sodium

JOSLIN EXCHANGES: 1 carbohydrate (1 fruit)

Prunes Poached in Red Wine and Lemon

A terrific end to a filling meal, these prunes are equally welcome at a leisurely Sunday brunch.

½ cup dry red wine such as California zinfandel (a good but not expensive red wine)
1 tablespoon brandy
1 teaspoon honey
2 2-inch strips lemon zest
1 small cinnamon stick
8 medium pitted prunes
2 tablespoons Crème Fraîche (page 224) or nonfat sugarless frozen vanilla yogurt
grated lemon zest for garnish (optional)

In a small saucepan, heat the wine, brandy, honey, lemon zest, and cinnamon stick to a boil. Add the prunes and bring to a boil again. Lower the heat and simmer for

10 minutes. Remove from the heat and let the prunes sit in the wine mixture until ready to serve. Do not chill.

To serve, place 4 prunes in each of 2 dessert dishes. Drizzle 1½ tablespoons of the wine liquid over the prunes. Top each serving with 1 tablespoon of crème fraîche. Top with grated lemon zest if desired.

Makes 2 servings.

PER SERVING: 143 calories (3% calories from fat), <1 g total fat (trace saturated fat), 2 g protein, 29 g carbohydrates, 5 g dietary fiber, 1 mg cholesterol, 15 mg sodium

JOSLIN EXCHANGES: 2 carbohydrate (2 fruit)

Strawberry Soufflés

You'll be surprised at how easy it is to make these individual soufflés. The recipe can easily be doubled to wow friends or, better yet, relatives. You'll need two ¾-cup individual soufflé cups or ovenproof baking dishes to make this recipe. ❡ If you have a few extra calories to spend, make a sauce out of sugar-free, fat-free vanilla pudding, thinning it with a bit of extra skim milk to make a crème anglaise. Open the cooked soufflé with two spoons in the middle of the top and add with a tablespoon of the vanilla sauce. Check the Joslin Exchanges (page 249) for additional exchanges.

butter-flavored cooking spray
1 cup quartered fresh strawberries that have been washed and hulled
2 teaspoons cornstarch dissolved in 2 teaspoons water
2 teaspoons sugar
1 egg white
⅛ teaspoon cream of tartar
2 tablespoons egg substitute

Preheat the oven to 375°F. Lightly coat the soufflé dishes with cooking spray and set aside.

Puree the fruit in a food processor or blender, leaving some small pieces of fruit intact. Transfer the fruit to a small nonstick saucepan. Stir in the dissolved cornstarch and sugar. Cook over medium heat for 2 to 3 minutes, until the mixture thickens. Remove from the heat.

Beat the egg white and cream of tartar with an electric mixer until stiff but not dry.

Add the egg substitute very slowly to the fruit, stirring so that the mixture does not curdle. Stir ¼ of the beaten egg white into the fruit to lighten the mixture. Fold in the rest of the egg whites until incorporated. Spoon the fruit mixture into the

prepared soufflé cups, dividing equally. Bake for about 15 minutes, until the soufflés are puffed and browned. Serve at once.

Makes 2 servings.

PER SERVING: 73 calories (10% calories from fat), 1 g total fat (0.1 g saturated fat),
4 g protein, 13 g carbohydrates, 1 g dietary fiber, <1 mg cholesterol, 56 mg sodium

JOSLIN EXCHANGES: ½ very low fat protein, 1 carbohydrate (1 fruit)

Ricotta-Stuffed Pears

The Italians have a tradition of combining wine, cheese, and fruit. Here is a delicious
way to end a meal. It also makes a nice salad on a bed of salad greens when the graham cracker topping is omitted. You can substitute pear halves packed in natural juice
for the fresh pear with good results.

> *1 teaspoon currants*
> *½ teaspoon Marsala or dry sherry*
> *1 large firm, ripe Bartlett or Anjou pear, cut in half and cored*
> *juice of ½ lemon*
> *1 tablespoon part-skim ricotta cheese*
> *1 tablespoon fat-free cream cheese*
> *⅛ teaspoon sugar substitute*
> *1 teaspoon graham cracker crumbs*

Place the currants and Marsala in a cup and set aside.

Cut a thin slice from the bottom of each pear half so that it will sit upright on
a plate. Rub the halves with lemon juice and place on dessert plates.

In a small bowl, combine the ricotta, cream cheese, and sugar substitute. Stir
in the wine and currants, and mix well. Divide the cheese mixture between the
pear halves, mounding in the hollow of the core. Sprinkle with the graham cracker
crumbs and serve at once.

Makes 2 servings.

PER SERVING: 98 calories (10% calories from fat), 1 g total fat (0.4 g saturated fat),
3 g protein, 21 g carbohydrates, 3 g dietary fiber, 3 mg cholesterol, 58 mg sodium

JOSLIN EXCHANGES: 1 carbohydrate (1 fruit)

APPENDIX 1

Two Weeks of Menus for 1,200 and 1,800 Calories

1,200-CALORIE MEAL PLAN	DAY 1	DAY 2	DAY 3
BREAKFAST ½ **nonfat milk** 1 **fruit** 1 **bread** 1 **meat** **Total Carbohydrate** **37 g**	4 oz nonfat milk Breakfast Banana Split	4 oz nonfat milk ¼ canteloupe Baked Cheese Grits	4 oz nonfat milk ½ grapefruit Oven-Baked Potato Pancakes with Yogurt and Applesauce scrambled egg
LUNCH 1 **vegetable** 1 **fat** 1 **fruit** 1 **bread** 2 **meat** **Total Carbohydrate** **30–35 g**	Tabbouleh in Romaine Leaves 2 oz Stuffed Burger	Roasted Zucchini with Yogurt Tuna and Pineapple on Peasant Bread	Pichi Pachi sprinkled with 3 T Parmesan cheese
SNACK ½ **milk** 1 **bread** **Total Carbohydrate** **22 g**	4 oz nonfat yogurt apple	4 oz nonfat milk blueberries	1 oz low-fat cheese 6 saltines
DINNER ½ **milk** 2 **vegetable** 1 **fat** 2 **bread** 2 **meat** **Total carbohydrate** **37–47 g**	Broccoli and Red Pepper Salad Chicken Tacos	tossed salad and 2 T low-fat dressing Swordfish Kebabs	Roasted Cauliflower Parmesan Snapper Stew with New Potatoes and Tomatoes

DAY 4	DAY 5	DAY 6	DAY 7
			8 oz nonfat yogurt
			½ peach
fresh grapes	½ cup fresh fruit cocktail		
Chile Relleno Casserole	Cinnamon-Raisin Puffed French Toast	Cheese Blini with Strawberries	Orange-Scented Brown Rice with Peaches and Milk
tossed salad with nonfat dressing			
1/16 honeydew	pear with 4 oz fruited yogurt		
Turkey Tortilla Roll-ups	Veggie Sandwich	White Bean, Spinach, and Red Pepper Soup 1 oz low-fat cheese	Sausage and Mush-room Pizza
3 cups popcorn with 3 T Parmesan cheese	4 oz nonfat milk 1½ low-fat cream-filled cookie	1 T peanut butter on toast	Roasted Pineapple, Margarita Style, with 4 oz plain nonfat yogurt
salad with nonfat dressing		4 oz nonfat milk Beet and Orange Salad ½ cup Couscous with Currants and Wal-nuts	salad with nonfat dressing
Rotini with Eggplant, Tomatoes, and Ricotta Cheese or 3 T Parmesan cheese	Cajun Grilled Chicken on Yellow Rice and Peas	½ serving Turkey Stroganoff	Linguine with Easy Clam Sauce

1,200-CALORIE MEAL PLAN

	DAY 1	DAY 2	DAY 3
BREAKFAST **½ milk** **1 fruit** **1 bread** **1 meat** **Total Carbohydrate 37 g**	4 oz nonfat milk Blueberry Scone 1 oz Mini Babybel Bonbel low-fat cheese	 2 slices whole wheat toast Egg Florentine	4 oz nonfat milk 2 slices Canadian Bacon Spoon Bread
LUNCH **1 vegetable** **1 fat** **1 fruit** **1 bread** **2 meat** **Total Carbohydrate 30–35 g**	Warm Spinach Salad Frozen Gelatin Mousse pita pocket	 fresh strawberries Individual Cheesecake Shrimp Gazpacho	 Lentils and Cheese in Pita 4 oz nonfat milk
SNACK **½ milk** **1 bread** **Total Carbohydrate 22 g**	½ banana with 4 oz nonfat yogurt	fat-free tortilla chips with salsa and 1 oz low-fat melted cheese	low-fat granola with 4 oz nonfat milk
DINNER **½ milk** **2 vegetable** **1 fat** **2 bread** **2 meat** **Total Carbohydrate 37 g**	4 oz nonfat milk ½ serving Mediterranean Salad Gingered Chicken Soup Blackberry Cobbler	½ serving Cucumber, Sweet Onion, and Cherry Tomato Salad Old-Fashioned Bread Pudding Barbecued Clams and Mussels	 Strawberry Soufflé Fresh Tomato Basil Pizza

DAY 4	DAY 5	DAY 6	DAY 7
Breakfast Pizza	⅛ honeydew melon Low-Fat Granola Muffin Creole Egg Casserole	strawberries with yogurt Open-Faced Breakfast Sandwich	4 oz nonfat milk Baked Apples with Yogurt and Almonds 1 oz low-fat cheese
Quick Roasted Plum Tomatoes Simply Delicious Black Beans	tossed salad with dressing banana slices ½ serving Stuffed Pasta Shells	tossed salad with nonfat dressing Green Beans with Almonds and Balsamic Vinegar Low-Fat Macaroni and Cheese 4 oz nonfat milk	Jicama Slaw fresh peach Grilled Chicken Salad with Summer Salsa Dressing
4 oz nonfat milk 1 oz pretzels	Ricotta-Stuffed Pear	4 oz nonfat milk ¾ cup cereal	4 oz nonfat milk 1 Dried Apricot Scone
Snow Pea Salad Apple Tart Orange Roughy Baked in Foil	Grilled Vegetable Skewers ½ serving Lemon Rice with Dried Apricots ½ serving Broiled Sole with Lemon, Tomato, and Capers	steamed broccoli Easy Fried Rice Roasted Pork Tenderloin	4 oz nonfat milk Green Beans with Herbs Crispy Garlic Potatoes ½ serving All-American Turkey Loaf

1,800-CALORIE MEAL PLAN	DAY 1	DAY 2	DAY 3
BREAKFAST ½ milk 1 fruit 2 bread 1 fat 1 meat **Total Carbohydrate** **52 g**	½ grapefruit ½ large bagel 2 T low-fat cream cheese Mushroom Omelet	½ serving fresh blue-berries Huevos Rancheros	peach halves Breakfast Burrito
LUNCH 2 vegetable 1 fat 2 bread 1 fruit 2 meat **Total Carbohydrate** **45–55 g**	Cobb Salad Bow Ties with As-paragus, Cherry Tomatoes, and Mush-rooms	Rice Stick Noodles and Spicy Vegetables ½ serving Grilled Cornish Hen, Thai Style	Tapioca Pudding with Berries 2 slices pineapple Mexicali Stuffed Pep-pers
SNACK ½ milk 1 fruit **Total Carbohydrate** **22 g**	5 melba toast and 1 oz low-fat cheese	4 oz nonfat milk and ¾ cup unsweetened cereal	6 vanilla wafers with ½ cup sugar-free pudding
DINNER ½ milk 3 vegetable 1 fat 3 meat 4 bread **Total Carbohydrate** **67–82 g**	4 oz nonfat milk Baked Asparagus with Lemon Bread Crumbs Scallops with Rotini and Pesto	Baked Ratatouille Turkey Scalloppine Marsala Crispy Garlic Pota-toes Prunes Poached in Red Wine and Lemon	4 oz nonfat milk Medley of Winter Roots Orange Roughy Baked in Foil ½ serving Dilled Rice with Baby Peas Old-Fashioned Bread Pudding
SNACK ½ milk 2 bread **Total Carbohydrate** **37 g**	2 slices raisin toast and ¼ cup low-fat ricotta cheese	½ cup nonfat milk Blueberry Scone	English muffin and 1 oz nonfat cheese

DAY 4	DAY 5	DAY 6	DAY 7
Bagel Thins with Smoked Salmon Cream Cheese	Silver Dollar Apple Pancakes with low-sugar pancake syrup ¼ cup nonfat cottage cheese	Breakfast Crepes	4 oz nonfat milk ¼ canteloupe Low-Fat Pumpkin Muffin scrambled egg
Broiled Tomatoes with Feta Cheese Meatless White Chili	salad with 2 T low-fat dressing Pasta with Black Beans 4 oz fruited yogurt	1/16 honeydew melon Roasted Vegetables over Fettuccine with 6 T grated Parmesan cheese	Mushroom Ravioli with Chunky Tomato Sauce fresh figs ½ serving Stuffed Burger
8 oz fruited nonfat yogurt with sugar substitute	15 Teddy Grahams with 4 oz nonfat milk	¼ cup Grape-Nuts with 4 oz plain nonfat yogurt	4 oz nonfat milk 1 cup bean soup
4 oz nonfat milk tossed greens and 2 T low-fat dressing Shrimp Fajitas Roasted Pineapple, Margarita Style	Roasted Cauliflower Parmesan Baked Salmon with Dill on Steamed Cabbage Lemon Rice with Dried Apricots	Chicken Curry Dilled Rice with Baby Peas Individual Ice Cream Bombe	4 oz nonfat milk Summer Vegetable Stir-Fry Broiled Cod with Warm Corn and Sweet Onion Relish Cajun Spiced Rice
20 nonfat tortilla chips and salsa with 1 oz mozzarella cheese	4 oz nonfat yogurt 6 gingersnaps	4 oz nonfat milk 4 breadsticks	6 cups popcorn with 3 T grated Parmesan cheese

1,800-CALORIE MEAL PLAN	DAY 1	DAY 2	DAY 3
BREAKFAST ½ **milk** **1 fruit** **2 bread** **1 fat** **1 meat** Total Carbohydrate 52 g	4 oz nonfat milk 2 oz orange juice Creamy Polenta with Dried Fruits 1 oz low-fat cheese	pear slices 1 slice low-calorie whole wheat bread Texas Chicken Sausage Patties with Grits	8 oz nonfat yogurt 1 T raisins Homemade Muesli
LUNCH **2 vegetable** **1 fat** **2 bread** **1 fruit** **2 meat** Total Carbohydrate 45–55 g	2 slices pineapple Swordfish Kebabs	½ serving Caesar Salad with Grilled Tuna orange segments	Vegetable Soup with Rice ½ whole wheat bun ½ serving Turkey Cutlets with Warm Fruit Relish
SNACK ½ **milk** **1 fruit** Total Carbohydrate 22 g	Fruit shake: 4 oz non-fat milk, ½ banana, 2–3 ice cubes; blend until smooth	Stuffed potato: 1 small baked potato and 1 oz melted cheese 1 broccoli spear, steamed and chopped	4 oz plain nonfat yogurt 3 gingersnaps
DINNER ½ **milk** **3 vegetable** **1 fat** **3 meat** **4 bread** Total Carbohydrate 67–82 g	4 oz nonfat milk Green Beans with Almonds and Balsamic Vinegar Grilled Turkey Burger with Pineapple Kasha with Zucchini	4 oz nonfat milk tossed salad with nonfat dressing Low-Fat Macaroni and Cheese	½ serving Mediterranean Salad Lemon Veal with Mushrooms and Capers 2 servings Red Potato Salad
SNACK ½ **milk** **2 bread** Total Carbohydrate 37 g	medium baked potato with 1 oz melted low-fat cheese 1 broccoli spear	¼ cup nonfat cottage cheese 1½ oz pretzels	4 oz nonfat milk Dried Apricot Scone

DAY 4	DAY 5	DAY 6	DAY 7
Apple Bran Muffin Breakfast Cod with Grapefruit and Horseradish Sauce	4 oz nonfat milk ½ fruit cup Crustless Spinach Quiche ½ English muffin with 1 tsp margarine	Prunes Poached in Red Wine and Lemon Low-Fat Granola Muffin Creole Egg Casserole	6 oz nonfat milk Buttermilk Griddle Cakes with Sautéed Pears
⅓ cup steamed rice Fresh Fruit Cup Curried Tofu and Vegetables	Broccoli and Red Pepper Salad Ricotta-Stuffed Pears Baked Chicken Quesadilla	Cucumber, Sweet Onion, and Cherry Tomato Salad Blackberry Cobbler Turkey Tortilla Roll-up	Fresh pear Pichi Pachi
½ cup sugar-free custard 20 small pretzels	¼ cup low-fat cottage cheese 8 animal crackers	3 graham crackers and 1 T peanut butter	8 oz Alba sugar-free shake, with water
Stuffed Pasta Shells Baked Spiced Pears	Low-Fat Open-Faced Tuna Melt	Jicama Slaw Green Beans with Herbs Yogurt Cinnamon Chicken ½ serving Couscous with Currants and Walnuts Pineapple Upside-Down Cake	Linguine with Sautéed Garlic, Broccoli, and Mushrooms Easy Chicken Cacciatore with Summer Squash
Apple tart and 4 oz nonfat yogurt	½ cup sugar-free pudding 6 graham squares	½ cup Grape-Nuts and 4 oz nonfat yogurt	1 large pita with 1 oz water-packed tuna and 1 T nonfat mayo

APPENDIX 2

Medical Questions

Questions People with Diabetes Most Often Ask Their Health Care Team

My doctor says I have a "touch of sugar." Does this mean I have diabetes? Is it serious? What do I need to do about it?

Probably, yes. If your doctor reports that you have a "touch of sugar," you have probably been given a fasting plasma glucose test that showed a level in excess of 126 mg/dl (milligrams per deciliter), the number that indicates the presence of diabetes. The number had been lowered because people have few symptoms in the early stages of diabetes and may have elevated levels of glucose for seven years or longer before a diagnosis is made. During that time damage may have occurred in the body, including retinopathy, heart and vascular diseases, as well as kidney disease and neuropathy.

People who develop diabetes when they are over forty often have type 2 diabetes, although it can occur in younger people—especially those who are overweight. People with type 2 diabetes actually produce some insulin, but either it is not enough to meet their needs or for some reason it does not properly signal the cells to allow glucose to enter.

Untreated or poorly treated diabetes can cause life-threatening problems. A diagnosis of diabetes deserves immediate nutritional and medical intervention, along with a regimen of exercise. This three-pronged approach is the best way to minimize complications.

I've been to my doctor, and he gave me a diet. I don't eat some of the foods that are on the list. I don't really understand what an exchange is. Help!

All people with diabetes use different meal-planning approaches to control their diabetes. "Exchanges" is one of them. An exchange is merely a grouping of foods that are similar nutritionally. In the specific weights and amounts listed, each food on an exchange list is the same in terms of calories, protein, fat, and carbohydrate to every other food on that list. For example, all very low fat protein exchanges provide 35 to 45 calories, 7 grams of protein, 0 carbohydrate, and 0 to 2 grams of fat. Exchange lists provide a lot of variety. And since fruits, milk products, and starches have similar carbohydrate levels per serving, they can be substituted for one another, further expanding your food choices. (See Joslin Exchanges, page 249.)

The important thing is to eat a healthy, varied diet planned by a dietitian so your individual likes and dislikes can be taken into consideration.

What is carbohydrate counting? Why and how will this meal-planning approach help control my diabetes? Having diabetes means that I have to avoid eating sugar, right?

Carbohydrate counting is another meal-planning approach. Carbohydrates are those foods that enter the bloodstream exclusively as glucose shortly after we eat. Protein and fat contribute significantly less glucose to the bloodstream—almost all comes from carbohydrate.

Think of how much easier it would be to control blood sugars if we counted the number of grams of carbohydrates in a meal before eating and then took the proper medicine or insulin, or increased our exercise and then monitored to see the effect and to note further changes needed to achieve our target goal. For our purposes, carbohydrates are: all fruits; starchy vegetables such as peas, corn, and root vegetables; grains and dried beans; dairy products except cheese; desserts; candy; and beers and wines. On the other hand, fats and proteins enter the bloodsteam more slowly and therefore have a delayed effect on blood sugar levels. Glucose from metabolized protein does not appear in the bloodstream for two to three hours, and fat intake has an effect on blood sugar six hours after eating. About half of the insulin we produce or take in a day should be used to cover the carbohydrates we eat, and the other half should be used to keep blood sugar levels controlled in between meals.

To count carbohydrates you'll need three things: a meal plan, carbohydrate information, and blood sugar monitoring records. Information on how many grams of carbohydrates are in the foods you eat can be found on food labels, in books, and on exchange lists. Be sure when you rely on labels that you note the serving size because if you eat less or more, you will have to modify the gram count. Supermarkets often sell carbohydrate counters, but you will find more than one book on the subject at a bookstore or your library. There are books that give gram counts for name-brand processed foods, fast foods, and generic foods, so no guessing is necessary. You can also use the Joslin Exchange list (page 249).

To determine your optimum daily carbohydrate intake you and your dietitian will need to know your desired weight, your total calorie needs, and your activity level. Your dietitian will then help you calculate the number of grams of carbohydrates you should eat each day. Then you can decide on how to apportion these during the day based on your food preferences and lifestyle, and how you choose to take your diabetes medicine.

Sugar per se is not the culprit in high blood sugar levels. It has never been the cause of diabetes, nor has avoiding sugar ever cured diabetes. Dietary sugar is only one of many types of carbohydrates that affect blood glucose levels. Dietary sugar has little nutritional value, however. It is also usually found in foods high in saturated fat and calories.

When at the market, read the labels carefully for their carbohydrate content. Discuss the use of sugar and high-sugar foods in your diet with your dietitian or diabetes educator so that you can develop a meal plan that fits desserts into your lifestyle. You will need to consider how to match your food with either medicine or exercise to meet a goal of better blood sugar control. For more information about carbohydrate counting and insulin adjustment, see *The Joslin Guide to Diabetes*.

Okay, I understand about carbohydrates, but what is the glycemic index that I have read about and how will understanding it help me?

The glycemic index provides some useful information to consider when trying to manage blood sugar, but it is too imprecise to use alone. The actual blood glucose rise can be affected by how fast one eats and the amount of fat, fiber, and protein eaten with the carbohydrate. Even the manner of cooking a food can affect the rise in blood glucose—for instance, whether the carbohydrate is eaten raw, cooked slightly, or overcooked.

By using the index, together with carbohydrate counting, exchanges, or other meal-planning tools, you can monitor your carbohydrate choices to help ensure better control of your after-meal glucose levels.

Since the 1970s, research has focused on sugar and its impact on blood glucose. The glycemic index is a rating from 1 to 100 that tells us how quickly a food will raise our blood sugar after we eat equal amounts of carbohydrate from different sources. The higher the number, the faster the rise; the lower the number, the slower the rise. For example, look at the index for these breakfast cereals: cornflakes (83), All-Bran (54), oatmeal (53). With this information how would you change your choice of breakfast cereal? You may want to select All-Bran rather than cornflakes to help decrease the rise in your blood sugar. Remember that it is not only what you eat but how much. For example, note the relatively low index for oatmeal. Think about that index and the grams of carbohydrate you would be ingest-ing if you ate 1½ cups (45 grams of carbohydrate) rather than ½ cup (15 grams of carbohydrate).

Can you send me a diabetic diet or give me a list of menus for a week or two that I can follow?

There is no such thing as a "diabetic diet." Following a carefully developed nutri-tion program can help you consistently distribute the nutrients you need to eat for good health every day. You and your dietitian will need to develop a meal plan that takes into account

- your goals. Do you need to lose weight, gain weight, or maintain your cur-rent weight?
- your medication. Are you taking insulin or oral medications? If so, how much and when does the action of your medication peak?
- your medical condition. Do you have other medical problems such as high blood lipids (fats in the blood) or kidney disease that may influence what you should or should not eat?
- your lifestyle preferences. What kinds of food do you like and dislike? Are you a vegetarian? When do you exercise?

Beginning on page 231 you will find two weeks of sample menus, using recipes from this book, for three meals a day from Monday to Friday for people on 1,200-calorie-per-day and 1,800-calorie-per day meal plans. The Saturday and Sunday meal plans give suggestions for entertaining, either a weekend brunch or lunch or dinner with guests. Your dietitian or diabetes educator will help you incorporate these menus into your individual meal plan.

Your individual meal plan will be designed to keep blood sugars in a near-normal range while at the same time giving you freedom to choose the foods you want to eat. Your dietitian will also recommend that you eat foods low in saturated fat, cholesterol, and sodium.

Do you have a recipe for a birthday cake for someone with diabetes?

A birthday cake as well as other favorite foods can be worked into your meal plan. The challenge of "special occasions" and diabetes is how to indulge without the guilt and have good blood sugar control. Ask yourself these questions:

- Is it something I want to work into my plan?
- Do I need to adjust my insulin or medication or exercise?
- Is it made with heart-healthy fats?

You can indulge by planning a response. If it's a daily occurrence, more work may need to be done.

Below is a wonderfully tasty basic sponge cake that can serve as a great special-occasion dessert. You can have your cake and eat it, too! Adjust your insulin, medicine, and/or exercise for a more flexible meal plan.

BASIC SPONGE CAKE (GÉNOISE)

> *butter-flavored cooking spray*
> *2 cups sifted cake flour*
> *¾ cup fructose*
> *1 tablespoon baking powder*
> *½ teaspoon salt (optional)*
> *⅓ cup canola oil*
> *2 large eggs, separated*
> *½ cup egg substitute*
> *½ cup water*
> *1½ teaspoons vanilla extract*
> *grated zest of 1 lemon, 1 orange, or a combination (optional)*
> *1 cup egg whites (the whites from the 2 eggs plus 6 or 7 more), at room*
> *   temperature*
> *½ teaspoon cream of tartar*

Preheat the oven to 325°F. Lightly coat two 9-inch round cake pans or one 10-inch tube pan with cooking spray. Dust with flour.

In a large bowl, sift together the cake flour, fructose (that has been whirled in a food processor for 10 seconds), baking powder, and salt (if using). Make a well in the center. Beat together the canola oil, egg yolks, egg substitute, water, vanilla extract, and lemon zest. Pour into the flour mixture and blend well. In a large mixing bowl, beat the egg whites until frothy. Add the cream of tartar and beat until the egg whites form stiff peaks.

Stir about ½ cup of beaten egg whites into the flour and egg mixture to lighten it. Gently fold in the remaining egg whites. When thoroughly blended, divide the batter between the prepared cake pans. Bake for 25 to 30 minutes (50 to 55 minutes for the tube pan), until the cake is golden brown and begins to pull away slightly from the sides. *Do not* open the oven door until the cake is almost done, or it may fall. Run the spatula around the edges and turn out at once onto a wire rack. Cool completely. The cake can be made ahead, wrapped well, and frozen for up to 1 month.

Makes 16 servings.

PER SERVING: 144 calories (37% calories from fat), 6 g total fat (1 g saturated fat), 4 g protein, 19 g carbohydrate, trace dietary fiber, 27 mg cholesterol, 208 mg sodium

JOSLIN EXCHANGES: 1 carbohydrate (1 bread/starch), 1 fat

CHOCOLATE BUTTERCREAM FROSTING

1 cup fructose
6 tablespoons skim milk
4 tablespoons cornstarch
4 tablespoons unsweetened cocoa powder
2 large egg yolks
1 teaspoon vanilla extract
1 teaspoon salt (optional)
8 tablespoons cold unsalted butter
8 tablespoons cold stick margarine

In a medium saucepan, combine the fructose, skim milk, cornstarch, and cocoa powder. Bring to a boil, stirring constantly. Remove from the heat and stir until smooth and thick, about 3 minutes.

Using an electric mixer, beat the egg yolks, vanilla extract, and salt (if using). Add the butter and margarine, 1 tablespoon at a time, beating after each addition, until the frosting has the consistency of whipped butter. Use to frost 1 cake, using about ½ cup between the 2 layers and the remaining frosting on the sides and top. Refrigerate until ready to serve.

Makes about 2 cups, 16 servings

PER SERVING: 192 calories (56% calories from fat), 12 g total fat (3.5 g saturated), trace protein, 20 g carbohydrate, trace dietary fiber, 32 mg cholesterol, 104 mg sodium

JOSLIN EXCHANGES: 2 carbohydrate (2 bread/starch), 2 fat

I am having someone who has diabetes over to my house for dinner. What can I serve?

Everyone, including those who do not have diabetes, should be eating a diet low in saturated fat, cholesterol, and sodium. If you keep this in mind when planning your menu, it will be possible for the person with diabetes to enjoy your meal with few alterations. You can set aside small portions of the food—meat without the sauce, vegetables without the butter, salad without the dressing, and so forth.

Also important for a person with diabetes is the timing of the meal and the portion sizes. Discuss with your guest what his or her needs are and try to avoid any delays. Have low-calorie snacks available should an unexpected delay occur.

Are there any special minerals and vitamins I can take for diabetes?

If you are eating a balanced diet—the whole idea behind a meal plan—it is unlikely that you will need to take special vitamin or mineral supplements. However, recent medical studies have shown that certain vitamins, particularly C and E, may help prevent some of the long-term complications of diabetes such as nerve disorders, blood vessel disease, eye cataracts, and retinopathy. In some people other medical conditions or treatments may affect their mineral balance, which will then affect their diabetes.

New guidelines based on adequate mineral intake rather than recommended daily allowance were published in August 1997. Labels will begin to change, so it is more important than ever to read food labels carefully. Remember: Guidelines are based on healthy adults, and as a person with diabetes, your needs may differ. Check with your health care team before taking any vitamin or mineral supplement.

My doctor told me that I have high cholesterol. Does this mean I can't eat eggs?

Not exactly. There is more to the story. To reduce the risk of cardiovascular disease, everyone should limit cholesterol to less than 300 milligrams per day. One large egg contains 213 milligrams of cholesterol, all in the egg yolk. So while you can eat the egg white, you should limit egg yolks to no more than three per week and avoid fatty red meats and whole milk dairy products. To further lower your cholesterol level, you should eat more foods that are high in fiber, low in saturated as well as total fat, and naturally cholesterol free, such as fruits, vegetables, grains, pasta, dried beans, and bran. When cooking, use nonstick cooking sprays or a small amount of reduced-fat margarine in a nonstick pan. Avoid lard, bacon fat, and shortening. It's also important to keep your blood sugars under control because high blood sugars increase LDLs (low-density lipoproteins, which deposit cholesterol in the arteries) and decrease HDL (high-density lipoproteins, which sweep cholesterol out of the arteries).

I have a varied schedule and can never find time to eat right. How can I possibly manage my disease? How do I cope with late meals when entertaining or going out?

With the introduction of flexibility as an option in the control of diabetes, it is more important for you and your health care team to problem-solve concerning unusual situations.

Here are some options to accommodate late meals or dining out:

- decreased food at the meal
- increased exercise after the meal
- medication adjustment or additions
- no change because it happens infrequently

It doesn't require a lot of time or special talent to prepare quick, nourishing meals that will fit into your meal plan. What it does take, however, is some rethinking about how and what you cook. Enjoy your journey to better control of your diabetes by using this cookbook.

What is hypoglycemia, and how do I control it? Why am I sometimes unaware that my blood sugar is low?

A blood sugar below 60 mg/dl (milligrams per deciliter) means you have low blood sugar (hypoglycemia). Some people call it a reaction. You can *usually* tell that you have low blood sugar by the way you feel. The type and combination of reactions depends on the speed and severity of the fall of blood glucose levels. The most common symptoms are: confusion, silliness, numbness of lips, blurred vision, sweating, shaking, headache, tiredness, nausea, irritability, hunger, and fast heart rate.

Low blood sugar can occur rapidly. Friends or family may become aware of the change in your behavior before you are aware of the symptoms.

Reactions that occur while sleeping are somewhat different and include such symptoms as damp nightclothes and bed linens, restlessness, waking in the night with a fast heart rate, high blood sugar the next morning, loss of memory for words, headache or feeling "hung over" in the morning, and nightmares.

A word of caution to those who take insulin: Research has shown that having one reaction predisposes you to have another, and that second reaction will be harder to recognize.

If you have low blood sugar, you must treat it immediately. Failure to do so could cause more serious complications such as convulsions and unconsciousness.

The best treatment is carbohydrate. Fifteen grams of carbohydrate such as three glucose tablets, one tablespoon of honey, or three or four Sweettarts or Pixy Stix will quickly raise the blood sugar forty to sixty points. Wait fifteen minutes to be sure. If you have not seen a rise by that time, treat with another 15 grams of carbohydrate. If your next meal is delayed more than one hour, you will need to have a snack. Eating a complex carbohydrate or protein, such as a small glass of skim milk or small piece of cheese, will keep your blood sugar from dropping later on. It is hard not to overeat when treating low blood sugar because you want to feel better. If you clean out your pantry or eat a box of chocolates, your weight goal may not be reached with all those extra calories. Have your glucose tablets with you at all times, and learn your symptoms and how to treat them.

Share with friends that you have diabetes so they can help if you do not recognize your symptoms. It is important for anyone who experiences low blood sugar to evaluate why. You may need to modify your medication and meal plan as your schedule changes.

Hypoglycemia unawareness may be a problem. Some people with diabetes lose the ability to recognize falling blood sugar. It occurs more often the longer one has had diabetes because less of the stress hormones are released that trigger the symptoms of hypoglycemia. Drinking alcohol may also lead to this condition. Research shows that having one episode of low blood sugar often makes recognizing the next more difficult. The person who has frequent low blood sugar may not recognize that this condition exists and therefore may have to rely on others for help. If bizarre, irrational, and angry behavior accompanies the insistence that you feel fine, you may have this condition. The treatment goal may be to keep blood sugar slightly higher so as to avoid frequent hypoglycemia. Or, taking a course in blood glucose awareness training may be the answer.

Your health care team will be of great help in figuring out what is happening and how to control low blood sugar. Testing your blood sugar during the night will be required to determine the action of your bedtime insulin. Rethinking the day, reviewing the time that you ate or exercised and took medication, can help you better understand trends. Blood glucose awareness training may be recommended.

APPENDIX 3

The Joslin Diabetes Exchange List for Meal Planning

The exchange categories that follow are different from those of a few years ago, because of a new understanding about how food is metabolized. Today, exchanges are grouped into Carbohydrates (bread/starch, fruit, milk, and vegetables—when consumed in sufficient quantities), Protein, and Fat. This new method for Exchanges allows for more individualized meal planning with your health care team, taking into account your lifestyle, food likes and dislikes, medical conditions, and goals.

Carbohydrates List

A carbohydrate serving (approximately 15 grams) may include a food choice from the fruit, milk, and starch categories. Vegetables are also carbohydrates but contain fewer grams of carbohydrate (5 grams) per serving, so if you are using carbohydrate counting as your meal-planning option, be sure to note the difference.

Carbohydrate Choices

Once choice provides:
Calories: 80
Protein: 3 g
Carbohydrate: 15 g
Fat: trace

Best choices: Whole grain breads and cereals, dried beans, and peas. (In general, one bread choice equals 1 oz of bread.)

Breads

ITEM	PORTION
White, whole wheat, rye, etc.	1 slice (1 oz)
Raisin, unfrosted	1 slice (1 oz)
Italian and French	1 slice (1 oz)
"Light" (1 slice equals 40 calories)	2 slices
Pita	
Pocket, 6-in. diameter	½ pocket
Mini size	1 pocket
Bagel	½ small (1 oz)
English muffin	½ small
Rolls	
Bulkie	½ small
Dinner, plain	1 small
Frankfurter	½ medium
Hamburger	½ medium
Bread crumbs	3 Tbsp.
Croutons	3 Tbsp.
Taco shells, small	2 (+ 1 Fat)
Tortilla, corn, 6-in. diameter	1
Tortilla, flour, 7-in. diameter	1 (+ 1 Fat)

Cereals

ITEM	PORTION
Cooked cereals	½ cup
Bran	
*All-Bran with extra fiber	1 cup
*All-Bran	⅓ cup

*Cereals high in fiber.

ITEM	PORTION
*100% bran	⅔ cup
*40% bran flakes	½ cup
*Bran Chex	½ cup
*Fiber One	⅔ cup
Multi-Bran Chex	⅓ cup
Cheerios	1 cup
Common Sense Oat Bran	½ cup
Corn or Rice Chex	¾ cup
Cornflakes	¾ cup
Crispix	½ cup
Fortified Oat Flakes	½ cup
Frosted flakes	⅓ cup
Granola, low-fat	¼ cup
Grape-Nuts	3 Tbsp.
*Grape-Nuts Flakes	⅔ cup
Just Right (with nuggets)	¼ cup
Kix	1 cup
Life	½ cup
Nutri-Grain	½ cup
Product 19	½ cup
Puffed rice or wheat	1½ cups
Rice Krispies	⅔ cup
*Shredded wheat biscuit	1 cup
Spoon size	½ cup
*Shredded Wheat 'n Bran	½ cup
Special K	1 cup
Team	⅔ cup
Total	¾ cup
*Wheat Chex	½ cup
*Wheaties	⅔ cup

Starchy Vegetables

ITEM	PORTION
Corn	½ cup
Corn on the cob	1 small
Lima beans	½ cup

*Cereals high in fiber.

ITEM	PORTION
Mixed vegetables, with corn or peas	⅔ cup
Parsnips	½ cup
Peas, green, canned or frozen	⅔ cup
Plantain, cooked	⅓ cup
Potato, white	
Mashed	½ cup
Baked	½ medium or 1 small (3 oz)
Sweet potato	
Mashed	⅓ cup
Baked	½ small or ½ cup (2 oz)
Pumpkin	¾ cup
Winter squash, acorn or butternut	¾ cup

Pasta (cooked)

ITEM	PORTION
Macaroni, noodles, spaghetti	½ cup

Legumes

ITEM	PORTION
Beans, peas, lentils (cooked)	½ cup
Baked beans, canned, no pork (vegetarian-style)	⅓ cup

Grains

ITEM	PORTION
Barley, cooked	⅓ cup
Bulgur, cooked	⅓ cup
Cornmeal	2½ Tbsp.
Cornstarch	2 Tbsp.
Couscous, cooked	⅓ cup
Flour	3 Tbsp.
Kasha, cooked	⅓ cup
Millet, dry	3 Tbsp.
Rice, cooked	⅓ cup
Wheat germ	¼ cup = 1 carb + 1 low fat protein

Crackers

Best choices: Lower-sodium products, i.e. saltines with unsalted tops.

ITEM	PORTION
AK-mak, regular and sesame	4 crackers
Animal crackers	8
Cheese Nips, reduced fat	22
Club, reduced fat	6
Finn Crisp	4
Gingersnaps	3
Graham crackers, 2½-in. squares	3
Granola bar, low-fat plain	1
Matzoh or matzoh with bran	1 (¾ oz)
Manischewitz whole wheat matzoh crackers	7
Melba toast rectangles	5
Melba toast rounds	10
Popcorn: popped, no fat added	3 cups
Orville Redenbacher Smart Pop!	4 cups
†Pretzels	7 regular or 12 mini
†Mr. Phipps pretzel chips	12
Rice cakes, popcorn cakes	2
Mini rice cakes	8
Ry-Krisp, triple crackers	3
†Saltines	6
Social Tea	4
†Snack chips:	
Baked potato or tortilla chips	15 small or 8 large (¾ oz)
SnackWell's, fat-free:	
†Cheddar	24
†Cracked pepper	8
†Wheat	6
Stella D'oro Almond Toast	2
Stella D'oro Egg Biscuit	2
Stoned Wheat Thins	3
Today's Choice water crackers	5
Town House, reduced fat	8

†High in sodium.

ITEM	PORTION
Triscuits, reduced fat	5
Uneeda	4
Wasa Lite or Golden Rye or Hearty Rye crispbread	2

Crackers for Occasional Use

(Equal to one starch **plus** one fat choice)

ITEM	PORTION
Arrowroot	4
†Butter crackers	
Rounds	7
Rectangular	6
†Cheez-It	27
†Cheese Nips	20
†Club or Town House crackers	6
†Combos	1 oz
†Escort crackers	5
Granola bar: plain, raisin, or peanut butter	1
Lorna Doone	3
†Meal Mates	5
†Oyster crackers	24
†Peanut butter sandwich crackers	3
Pepperidge Farm:	
Bordeaux cookies	3
†Goldfish	36
Popcorn, microwave light	4 cups
†Ritz	7
†Sociables	9
Stella D'oro Sesame Breadsticks	2
Stella D'oro Breakfast Treats	1
Stella D'oro Golden Bar	1
Stella D'oro Lady Stella Assortment	3
†Sunshine HiHo	6
Teddy Grahams	15
†Tidbits	21
†Triscuits	5
Vanilla wafers	6

†High in sodium.

Wasa Fiber Plus crispbread...4
Wasa Sesame or
    Breakfast crispbread...2
†Waverly Wafers 6
†Wheat Thins, reduced-fat 13

Fruit Choices

One choice provides: **Best choices:** Fresh whole fruit
Calories 60   **Be sure:** To choose fresh, frozen, or canned fruit
Protein: 0   packed in its own juice or water with no added
Carbohydrate: 15 g   sugar.
Fat: 0

ITEM	PORTION
Apple, 2-in. diameter	1 small
Apple, dried	4 rings
Applesauce, unsweetened	½ cup
Apricots	
Fresh	4 medium
Canned	4 halves
Dried	7 halves
Banana, 9-in. length, peeled	½
Banana flakes or chips	3 Tbsp.
Blackberries	¾ cup
Blueberries	¾ cup
Boysenberries	1 cup
Canned fruit, unless otherwise stated	½ cup
Cantaloupe, 5-in. diameter	
Sectioned	⅓ melon
Cubed	1 cup
Casaba, 7-in. diameter	
Sectioned	⅙ melon
Cubed	1⅓ cups
Cherries	
Sweet fresh	12
Dried (no sugar added)	2 Tbsp.
Cranberries, dried (no sugar added)	2 Tbsp.
Currants	2 Tbsp.

†High in sodium.

ITEM	PORTION
Dates	3
Figs	
Fresh	2 small
Dried	1 small
Granadillas (passionfruit)	4
Grapefruit, 4-in. diameter	½
Grapes	15 small
Guavas	1½ small
Honeydew melon, 6½-in. diameter	
Sectioned	⅛ melon
Cubed	1 cup
Kiwi (3 oz)	1 large
Kumquats	5 medium
Loquats, fresh	12
Lychees, fresh or dried	10
Mango	½ small
Sliced	½ cup
Nectarine, 2½-in. diameter	1 small
Orange, 3-in. diameter	1 small
Papaya, 3½-in. diameter	
Sectioned	½
Cubed	1 cup
Peach, 2½-in. diameter	1 small
Pear	1 small
Persimmon	
Native	2
Japanese, 2½-in. diameter	½
Pineapple	
Fresh, diced	¾ cup
Canned, packed in juice	⅓ cup
Plaintain, cooked	⅓ cup
Plums, 2-in. diameter	2 small
Pomegranate, 3½-in. diameter	½
Prunes, dried, medium	3
Raisins	2 Tbsp.
Raspberries	1 cup
Rhubarb, fresh, diced	3 cups
Strawberries, whole	1⅓ cups

Tangerines, 2½-in. diameter .... 2 small
Watermelon, diced .... 1¼ cups

Fruit Juice

Be sure to monitor your blood glucose: Fruit juice may elevate blood glucose rapidly, especially when consumed on an empty stomach or with a small amount of food such as a snack. Limit your intake of juice to no more than one meal each day or to times when you are engaging in vigorous activity or treating a low blood sugar.

ITEM	PORTION
Apple juice, unsweetened	4 oz
Cranapple, unsweetened	3 oz
Cranberry, unsweetened	4 oz
Cranberry, low-calorie	9 oz
Grape juice, unsweetened	3 oz
Grapefruit juice, unsweetened	5 oz
Lemon juice	8 oz
Orange juice, unsweetened	4 oz
Pineapple juice, unsweetened	4 oz
Prune juice, unsweetened	3 oz
Twister Light (with aspartame)	15 oz
Twister, regular	4 oz

Vegetable Choices

One choice provides:
Calories: 25
Protein: 2 g
Carbohydrate: 5 g
Fat: 0

Best choices: Fresh or raw vegetables: dark green, leafy, or orange.

Be sure: To choose at least 2 vegetables each day.

We encourage: Steaming with a minimum amount of water. Portion listed is for **cooked** serving unless noted otherwise.

ITEM	PORTION
Artichoke	½
Asparagus	1 cup
Bamboo shoots	1 cup
Bean sprouts	½ cup
Beets	½ cup
Beet greens	½ cup
Broccoli	½ cup

ITEM	PORTION
Brussels sprouts	½ cup
Cabbage	1 cup
Carrots	½ cup
Cauliflower	1 cup
Celery	1 cup
Collard greens	1 cup
Eggplant	½ cup
Fennel leaf	1 cup
Green beans	1 cup
Green pepper	1 cup
Kale	½ cup
Kohlrabi	½ cup
Leeks	½ cup
Mushrooms, fresh	1 cup
Mustard greens	1 cup
Okra	½ cup
Onion	½ cup
Pea pods, Chinese (snow peas)	½ cup
Radishes	1 cup
Red pepper	1 cup
Rutabagas	½ cup
†Sauerkraut	½ cup
Spinach	½ cup
Squash	
Summer	1 cup
Spaghetti	½ cup
Zucchini	1 cup
Swiss chard	1 cup
Tomato (ripe)	1 medium
†Tomato, canned	½ cup
Tomato juice or V8 juice	½ cup
†Tomato paste	1½ Tbsp.
Tomato sauce, canned	⅓ cup
Spaghetti sauce, jar	¼ cup
Turnip greens	1 cup

†These vegetables are high in sodium (salt). Low-sodium vegetables, juices, and sauces should be purchased if you are following a sodium-restricted diet. Fresh and frozen vegetables are lower in sodium than canned vegetables, unless the canned product states "low sodium."

Turnips..½ cup
Vegetables, mixed..½ cup
Wax beans..½ cup
Water chestnuts...............................6 whole or ¼ cup

Because of their low carbohydrate and calorie content, the following **raw** vegetables may be used liberally:

Alfalfa sprouts   Lettuce, all types
Celery   Mushrooms
Chicory   Parsley
Chinese cabbage   †Pickles (unsweetened)
Cucumber   Pimiento
Endive   Spinach
Escarole   Watercress

Milk Choices

Best choices: Nonfat or low-fat
Be sure: You take calcium supplements if you use less than 2 cups per day for adults, 3–4 cups per day for children.

Nonfat Selections
One choice provides:
Calories: 90
Protein: 8 g
Carbohydrate: 12 g
Fat: 0

ITEM	PORTION
Nonfat milk (skim)	1 cup
Nonfat buttermilk	1 cup
½% milk	1 cup
Nonfat plain yogurt	¾ cup
Nonfat yogurt made with Aspartame, i.e. Yoplait Light, Weight Watchers Ultimate 90 Dannon Light	6–8 oz
Lactaid milk (skim)	1 cup

†These vegetables are high in sodium (salt).

ITEM	PORTION
Powdered, nonfat milk, dry	⅓ cup
Canned, evaporated skim milk	½ cup
‡Sugar-free hot cocoa mix plus 6 oz of water	1 cup

Low-Fat Selections

One choice provides:

Calories: 105
Protein: 8 g
Carbohydrate: 12 g
Fat: 3 g

ITEM	PORTION
1% milk	1 cup
1% buttermilk	1 cup
Yogurt, plain, unflavored	¾ cup
Lactaid milk (1%)	1 cup

Medium- and High-Fat Selections

One choice provides:

Calories: 120–150
Protein: 8 g
Carbohydrate: 12 g
Fat: 5–8 g

The following milk items should be used sparingly due to their high saturated fat and cholesterol content.

ITEM	PORTION
2% milk	1 cup
Whole milk	1 cup

‡Most cocoa mixes do not provide the same amount of calcium as one cup of milk. Mixes which do provide the same amount should indicate on the label that the product contains 30% Daily Value for calcium. An example of a product which meets these calcium requirements is Alba sugar-free hot cocoa mix.

Other Carbohydrates

Breakfast Items

ITEM	PORTION	FOOD GROUP	GRAMS CARB	CAL
Nutri-Grain bar	1	2 carbs + 1 fat	27 g	205
Muffin, bran or corn	small (2 oz)	1 carb + 1 fat	22 g	125
Muffin, from mix	1/12 of pkg.	1 carb + 1 fat	17 g	125
Weight Watchers blueberry muffin	1	2 carbs + 1 fat	33 g	205
Croissant	1 (2 oz)	2 carbs + 2 fat	25 g	250
Doughnut, cake-type	1 small (1 oz)	1 carb + 1 fat	12 g	125
Doughnut, frosted	1 (2 oz)	2 carbs + 2 fat	30 g	250
Sweet roll/danish	1 (2 oz)	2 carbs + 2 fat	28 g	250
Biscuit	1 (1 oz)	1 carb + 1 fat	13 g	125
Corn bread, from mix	1 (2 oz)	2 carbs + 1 fat	30 g	205
Pancake	2 (4-in. diam.)	1 carb	13 g	125
Waffle Homemade	4-in. diam.	1 carb + 0–1 fat	13 g	125
Frozen	4-in. diam.	1 carb + 1 fat	15 g	125
Granola Regular	1/4 cup	1 carb + 1 fat	20 g	125
Low-fat	1/4 cup	1 carb	16 g	80

Desserts

ITEM	PORTION	FOOD GROUP	GRAMS CARB	CAL
Angel food cake	1/12 of cake	2 carbs	30 g	160
Brownie, unfrosted	2-inch square	2 carbs + 1 fat	25 g	205
Cake, unfrosted	2 oz	2 carbs + 1 fat	35 g	205
Cake, frosted	2 oz	3 carbs + 1 fat	40 g	285
Cookies: Fig Newtons, fat-free or regular	2	1 carb	22 g	80
SnackWell's fat-free: Creme-filled	2	1 carb	21 g	80
Chocolate truffle	1	1 carb	13 g	80
Devil's food or fudge	1	1 carb	13 g	80
Brownie	1	2 carbs	26 g	160

ITEM	PORTION	FOOD GROUP	GRAMS CARB	CAL
SnackWell's reduced-fat chocolate chip	15	1 carb	15 g	80
Cupcake, frosted	1	2 carbs + 1 fat	28 g	205
Ice cream (Edy's or Breyers):				
Regular	½ cup	1 carb + 2 fat	17 g	170
Low-fat or fat-free	½ cup	1 carb	22 g	80
No sugar added	½ cup	1 carb + 1 fat	15 g	125
Fat-free, no sugar added	½ cup	1 carb	19 g	80
Frozen dessert bars:				
Creamsicle, regular	1 bar	1 carb + 1 fat	19 g	125
Dole Fruit'n Cream Bar	1 bar	1 carb	17 g	80
Dole Fruit'n Juice Bar, regular	1 bar	1 carb	16 g	80
Eskimo Pie Pudding Bar	1 bar	1 carb	15 g	80
Häagen-Dazs fat-free Sorbet 'n' Yogurt	1 bar	1 carb	20 g	80
Fudgsicle fudge bar, No sugar added	2 bars	1 carb	16 g	80
Push-up	1 bar	1 carb	20 g	80
Welch's Fruit Juice Bar:				
Regular	1 bar	1 carb	11 g	80
No sugar added	2 bars	1 carb	12 g	80
Weight Watchers:				
Chocolate mousse bar	2 bars	1 carb	18 g	80
Orange Vanilla Treat	2 bars	1 carb	17 g	80
Ice cream sandwich	1	2 carbs + 1 fat	30 g	205
Frozen yogurt (Edy's or Breyers):				
Low-fat	½ cup	1 carb + 1 fat	17 g	125
Fat-free	½ cup	1 carb	22 g	80
Fat-free, no sugar added	½ cup	1 carb	18 g	80
Sherbet, sorbet	½ cup	2 carbs	27 g	160

ITEM	PORTION	FOOD GROUP	GRAMS CARB	CAL

Pudding:

| Sugar-free | ½ cup | 1 carb | 14 g | 80 |
| Regular | ½ cup | 2 carbs | 29 g | 160 |

Miscellaneous

ITEM	PORTION	FOOD GROUP	GRAMS CARB	CAL

Jam/jelly, honey, regular	1 Tbsp.	1 carb	13 g	80
Spaghetti sauce	½ cup	1 carb + 0–1 fat	10 g	125
Sugar	1 Tbsp.	1 carb	12 g	46

Syrup:

Light	2 Tbsp.	1 carb	13 g	80
Regular	2 Tbsp.	2 carbs	27 g	160
Yogurt, fruited, regular	1 cup	3 carbs	45 g	240

"Free" Foods List

Be sure: The following foods contain very few calories and may be used freely in your meal plan. Items marked with a dagger (†) are high in sodium; you should check with your doctor or dietitian before using these products.

General:

†Bouillon, broth, or consommé
Chewing gum, sugar-free
Cocoa powder
Coffee, tea
Cranberries (unsweetened)
Extracts
Gelatin mixes, sugar-free
Herbs, seasonings, spices
Lemon/lime juice
Lemon/lime/orange rind
Noncaloric diet soft drinks, unsweetened seltzer waters
†Pickles (unsweetened)
Postum (limit to 3 cups daily)
†Soy sauce, steak sauce

†Hot pepper sauce, taco sauce
Unprocessed bran (1 Tbsp.)
Vinegar

Many fat-free choices contain one or more types of sugar. The amount of sweetener is small; however, the portion used should be no more than the amount listed on this page or no more than *20 calories per serving,* approximately three times per day. Always read the labels carefully, and consult your physician or dietitian if you plan to use these items regularly.

Protein List

Best choices: Very low fat or low-fat selections.
Be sure: To trim off visible fat. Bake, broil, or steam selections with no added fat. Weigh your portion after cooking.
We encourage: Portions to be the accompaniment rather than the main course.

Very Low Fat Selections
One choice provides:
Calories: 35–45
Protein: 7 g
Carbohydrate: 0
Fat: 0–2 g

ITEM	PORTION
Beef:	
Healthy Choice 96% fat-free ground beef	1 oz
†Cheese products, fat-free:	
Kraft Free, Alpine Lace slices	1 slice
Healthy Choice or Kraft shredded	3 Tbsp.
†Cottage cheese, fat-free or 1%	¼ cup
†Ricotta, 100% fat-free	1 oz
Dried beans, cooked	½ cup = 1 protein + 1 carb
Egg substitute, plain	¼ cup
(less than 40 calories per serving)	

†High in sodium.

Egg whites...2

Poultry: chicken, turkey, or Cornish hen—

　　white meat only and skinless...1 oz

Fish and seafood: fresh or frozen cod, flounder, haddock,

　　halibut, trout, tuna (packed in water); clams, crab,

　　lobster, scallops, shrimp, imitation crabmeat ....1 oz

Game: venison, buffalo, ostrich ....1 oz

Ground turkey, 93–99% fat-free only ....1 oz

†Hot dogs, 97% fat-free ....1 oz

†Luncheon meats:

　　95% fat-free pastrami, ham, turkey ham, turkey bologna ....1 oz

†Turkey sausage, 97% fat-free...1 oz

Low-Fat Selections

One choice provides:

Calories: 55

Protein: 7 g

Carbohydrate: 0

Fat: 3 g

ITEM	PORTION
Beef:	
USDA Select or Choice grades of flank, round, sirloin, T-bone, tenderloin cuts	1 oz
ground beef, 90% fat-free	1 oz
†Cheeses:	
Cottage cheese, 4.5% fat	¼ cup
Mozzarella, light	1 oz
Kraft Light, slices:	1 oz
Fish:	
herring, uncreamed or †smoked	1 oz
Oysters, salmon, sardines (packed in tomato or mustard sauce†)	1 oz
Ground turkey or chicken, lean only	1 oz
†Hot dogs, 90% fat-free	1
†Luncheon meats, 90% fat-free	1 oz

†High in sodium.

ITEM	PORTION

Pork: lean only, center loin, fresh ham, loin chop, tenderloin.....1 oz
Poultry:
    Chicken or turkey, dark meat, no skin,
        or white meat with skin..1 oz
Tofu...3 oz
†Turkey sausage, 90% fat-free..1 oz
Veal: lean, trimmed only, loin chop, round ....1 oz

Medium-Fat Selections

One choice provides:
Calories: 75
Protein: 7 g
Carbohydrate: 0
Fat: 5 g

ITEM	PORTION

Beef: chipped, chuck, flank steak; hamburger (90% fat-free),
    rib eye, rump, sirloin, tenderloin top and bottom round.........1 oz
†Cheese:
    part-skim mozzarella, part-skim ricotta, farmer,
        Neufchâtel, Velveeta light, Jarlsberg Lite,
        Dorman's Slim Jack reduced-fat Monterey,
        Cracker Barrel light, Cabot light, Vitalait,
        Kraft Light ....1 oz
†Parmesan, Romano ....3 Tbsp.
‡Egg...1
Egg substitute with 60–80 calories per ¼ cup ....¼ cup
Lamb, except for breast...1 oz
†Luncheon meat, "light" (turkey bologna, turkey pastrami) ....1 oz
Peanut butter ....1 Tbsp. =
                                        1 protein + 1 fat
Pork, except for deviled ham, ground pork, and spare ribs ....1 oz
Turkey bacon..2 slices
Turkey franks, "light"..1 = 1½ protein
Veal, except for breast ....1 oz

†High in sodium.
‡Eggs are high in cholesterol. Limit consumption to 3 or 4 per week.

High-Fat Selections

One choice provides:
Calories: 100
Protein: 7 g
Carbohydrate: 0
Fat: 8 g

Be sure: Because of their high saturated fat and cholesterol content, the meat choices listed below should be used sparingly.

ITEM	PORTION

Beef:
    brisket, club and rib steak, *corned beef,
        regular hamburger with 20% fat, rib roast, short ribs ....1 oz
Cheese, regular:
    *blue, brie, cheddar, Colby, *feta, Monterey Jack,
        muenster, provolone, Swiss, *pasteurized process ....1 oz
Fish, fried..1 oz
Hot dog, regular, beef or pork ....1 oz = 1 protein + 1 fat
Lamb: breast ....1 oz
†Luncheon meats, regular: bologna, bratwurst,
    braunschweiger, knockwurst, liverwurst, pastrami,
    Polish sausage, salami ....1 oz
Organ meats:
    liver, heart, kidney...1 oz
Pork:
    †deviled ham, ground pork, spare ribs,
        *sausage (patty or link) ....1 oz
Poultry:
    capon, duck, goose..1 oz
Veal: breast...1 oz

Fat List

One choice provides:
Calories: 45
Protein: 0
Carbohydrate: 0
Fat: 5 g

Best choices: Monounsaturated fats. However, limit total amount of all types of fat.
Be sure: When using low-calorie version of fat choices, use amounts equal to 45 calories for one serving.

†High in sodium.

Monounsaturated Fats

ITEM	PORTION
Avocado, 4-in. diameter	⅛
Oils: canola, olive, peanut	1 tsp.
†Olives:	
Black	9 large
Green	10 large
Nondairy creamer:	
Liquid	2 Tbsp.
Reduced-fat liquid	5 Tbsp.
Nuts (unsalted):	
almonds	6
Brazil	2
cashews	6
filberts (hazelnuts)	5
macadamia	3
mixed	6
peanuts, Spanish	20
peanuts, Virginia	10
pecans	4 halves
pignolia (pine nuts)	1 Tbsp.
pistachio	12
Sesame seeds	1 Tbsp.
Tahini	2 tsp.

Polyunsaturated Fats

ITEM	PORTION
Margarine: stick, tub, or squeeze	1 tsp.
Reduced-fat	1 Tbsp.
Mayonnaise	1 tsp.
Reduced-fat	1 Tbsp.
Nuts: walnuts (unsalted)	4 halves
Oils: corn, cottonseed, safflower, soy, sunflower	1 tsp.
Salad dressings, regular:	
†French, 1,000 Island	1 Tbsp.
†Italian	2 tsp.

†High in sodium.

Creamy types ....2 tsp.
Salad dressings, reduced-calorie:
   †Italian...2 Tbsp.
   †Ranch...1 Tbsp.
   Red wine vinegar & oil ....2 Tbsp.
†Seeds: pumpkin, sunflower (unsalted) ....1 Tbsp.

Saturated Fats

ITEM	PORTION
†Bacon, cooked	1 strip
Butter:	
Stick	1 tsp.
Whipped	2 tsp.
Reduced-fat	1 Tbsp.
Chitterlings	2 Tbsp. (½ oz)
Coconut, shredded	2 Tbsp.
Coffee whitener, liquid	2 Tbsp.
Coffee whitener, powder	4 Tbsp.
Cream:	
Half & half	2 Tbsp.
Heavy	1 Tbsp.
Light	1½ Tbsp.
Whipped	1 Tbsp.
Whipped, pressurized	⅓ cup
Cream cheese:	
Regular	1 Tbsp.
Reduced-fat	2 Tbsp.
Oils: coconut or palm	1 tsp.
†Salt pork	¼ oz
Shortening or lard	1 tsp.
Sour cream:	
Regular	2 Tbsp.
Reduced-fat	3 Tbsp.

†High in sodium.

One choice = a free exchange

ITEM	PORTION
†Catsup	1 Tbsp.
Cream cheese:	
Philadelphia Free	1 Tbsp.
†Gravy:	
Pepperidge Farm 98% fat-free gravy	3 Tbsp.
Heinz HomeStyle fat-free gravy	¼ cup
Hard candy or mints, sugar-free	3 or less
Jams:	
Smucker's Light Preserves	1 Tbsp.
Smucker's Simply 100% Fruit	1 tsp.
Polaner All Fruit	1 tsp.
Knott's Berry Farm light preserves	1 Tbsp.
Mayonnaise:	
Cain's Fat-Free Mayonnaise	1 Tbsp.
Kraft Fat-Free Mayonnaise	2 Tbsp.
Kraft Miracle Whip Free	1 Tbsp.
Margarine:	
Fleischmann's fat-free squeeze bottle	¼ cup
Promise Ultra spread	2 tsp.
Promise Ultra, fat-free spread	¼ cup
Butter Buds	1 Tbsp.
Molly McButter	1 Tbsp.
Nonstick pan sprays	5-second spray
"I Can't Believe It's Not Butter" pump spray	5 sprays
†Mustard	1 Tbsp.
Frozen dessert bars, no sugar added:	
Fudgsicle	1 bar
Welch's Fruit Juice Bar	1 bar
Salad dressings:	
Good Seasons Fat-Free, all flavors:	2 Tbsp.
Kraft Free:	
Italian	2 Tbsp.
Ranch, Blue cheese	1 Tbsp.
1,000 Island, Catalina	1 Tbsp.

†High in sodium.

ITEM	PORTION

Seven Seas Free:
    Italian or Red Wine Vinegar ....2 Tbsp.
Wish-Bone Fat Free:
    Caesar, Creamy Roasted Garlic, Chunky Blue Cheese,
        French, 1,000 Island, Honey Dijon ....1 Tbsp.
Wish-Bone Lite:
    Italian or 1,000 Island ....2 Tbsp.
Hidden Valley:
    Blue Cheese ....2 Tbsp.
    Italian ....2 Tbsp.
    Caesar, Creamy Parmesan, Ranch, Honey Dijon ....1 Tbsp.
Sour cream, fat-free ....1 Tbsp.
Syrup:
    Cary's Sugar Free ....2 Tbsp.
    Fifty 50, reduced-calorie ....1 Tbsp.

Combination Foods List

Many foods are made up of several food groups. These mixed foods can be incorporated into your meal plan by substituting them for choices from more than one food group.

†Canned Soup

ITEM	PORTION	FOOD GROUP	GRAMS CARB	CAL
Rice or noodle with broth, prepared with water	8 oz	1 carb	9 g	80
Chunky styles, ready to serve	8 oz	1 carb, 1 protein	12 g	135
Cream soup: made with water	8 oz	1 carb, 1 fat	9 g	125

†High in sodium unless specially prepared without salt. Brands to look for that have less fat and sodium are:
Campbell's Healthy Request
Fantastic Foods (dried)
Healthy Choice
Progresso Healthy Classics

ITEM	PORTION	FOOD GROUP	GRAMS CARB	CAL
Made with 1% low-fat milk	8 oz	1 carb, 1 fat	15 g	125
Clam chowder, New England style prepared with 1% low-fat milk	8 oz	1 carb, 1 fat	20 g	125
Lentil with ham, ready to serve	8 oz	1 carb, 1 protein, 1 vegetable	20 g	160
Minestrone, ready to serve	8 oz	1 carb	16 g	80
Split pea with ham, ready to serve	8 oz	2 carb, 1 protein	28 g	215
Tomato, made with water	8 oz	1 carb	17 g	80
Vegetable, made with water	8 oz	1 vegetable	8 g	25

†Prepared Foods

ITEM	PORTION	FOOD GROUP	GRAMS CARB	CAL
Beef stew, homemade	1 cup	2 protein, 1 carb	15 g	190
Chicken pot pie, frozen	7 oz	2½ carb, 1 protein, 1 vegetable, 4 fat	40 g	460
Chili with meat and beans, homemade	1 cup	2 protein, 1 carb	22 g	190
Lasagna, homemade	2½ x 2½ x 1¾ in.	2 carb, 3 protein, 1 vegetable, 2 fat	35 g	215
Macaroni & cheese, made from package	1 cup	3 carb, 1 protein, 2 fat	45 g	385
†Pizza, cheese	⅛ of 14-in. diameter	1 carb, 1 protein, 1 vegetable, 1 fat	18 g	205

†High in sodium unless specially prepared without salt.

ITEM	PORTION	FOOD GROUP	GRAMS CARB	CAL
Ravioli,				
canned	1 cup (7 oz)	2 carb, 1 protein, 1 fat	30 g	260
*Spaghetti with meat,				
canned	1 cup	1 carb, 2 vegetable, 1 protein, 1 fat	26 g	230
†Spaghetti with meatballs,				
homemade	1 cup	2 carb, 2 protein	40 g	270
Taco,				
beef	1	2 protein, 1 carb, 1 fat	15 g	235

†High in sodium unless specially prepared without salt.

APPENDIX 4

Joslin Diabetes Center and Its Satellites and Affiliates

CONNECTICUT
Joslin Center for Diabetes at New Britain General Hospital
100 Grand Street
New Britain, CT 06050
(888) 4JOSLIN
(860) 224-5672

FLORIDA
Joslin Center for Diabetes at Morton Plant Mease Health Care
Clearwater, Dunedin, Countryside
455 Pinellas Street
Clearwater, FL 34616
(727) 461-8300

HAWAII
Joslin Center for Diabetes at Straub Clinic and Hospital
888 South King Street
Honolulu, HI 96813
(808) 522-4342

INDIANA
Floyd Memorial Hospital and Health Services
1850 State Street
New Albany, IN 47150
(812) 949-5700
(888) 77-FMHHS

MARYLAND
Joslin Center for Diabetes at University of Maryland Medical Center
22 South Greene Street
Baltimore, MD 21201-1595
(888) JOSLIN8

MASSACHUSETTS
Joslin Diabetes Center
One Joslin Place
Boston, MA 02215
(617) 732-2440

Joslin Center/Falmouth
210 Jones Road
Falmouth, MA 02540
(508) 548-1944

Joslin-Lahey Diabetes Center
1 Essex Center Drive
Peabody, MA 01960
(978) 538-4674

Joslin Center at Deaconess-Glover Hospital
148 Chestnut Street
Needham, MA 02192
(781) 453-5231

Joslin Center at Deaconess-Nashoba Hospital
200 Groton Road
Ayer, MA 01432
(978) 784-9534

Joslin Center at Deaconess-Waltham Hospital
5 Hope Avenue
Waltham, MA 02154
(781) 647-6222

NEW JERSEY
Joslin Center for Diabetes at St. Barnabas Ambulatory Care Centers
200 South Orange Avenue
Livingston, NJ 07039
(973) 325-6555

Joslin Center for Diabetes at Princeton
100 Canal Pointe Boulevard
Suite 100
Princeton, NJ 08540
(609) 987-0037

Joslin Center for Diabetes at St. Barnabas Medical Center
Community Medical Center
    Division
368 Lakehurst Road
Suite 305
Toms River, NJ 08753
(732) 349-5757

Joslin Center for Diabetes at Wayne General Hospital
410 Hamburg Turnpike
Suite 208
Wayne, NJ 07470
(201) 595-7100

NEW YORK
Joslin Center for Diabetes at St. Luke's– Roosevelt Hospital
425 West 59th Street
Suite 9C (Outpatient)
New York, NY 10019
(212) 523-8353

Joslin Center for Diabetes at SUNY Health Science Center
90 Presidential Plaza
Syracuse, NY 13202
(315) 464-5726

Joslin Center for Diabetes at Hudson Valley Hospital Center
222 Veterans Road
Suite 201
Yorktown Heights, NY 10598
(888) HVHC-JOSLIN
(914) 962-1320

PENNSYLVANIA
Joslin Center for Diabetes at Western Pennsylvania Hospital
5140 Liberty Avenue
Pittsburgh, PA 15224
(412) 578-1724

TENNESSEE
Joslin Center for Diabetes at Memorial Hospital
721 Glenwood Avenue
Suite West 461
Chattanooga, TN 37404
(423) 495-7970

WASHINGTON
Joslin Center for Diabetes at Swedish Medical Center (Outpatient Center)
910 Boylston Avenue
Seattle, WA 98104-0999
(206) 215-2440
(888) JOSLIN1

Metric Conversion Table

Liquid Measurements

¼ teaspoon = 1.25 milliliters
½ teaspoon = 2.5 milliliters
1 teaspoon = 5 milliliters
1 tablespoon = 15 milliliters
2 tablespoons = 30 milliliters
¼ cup = 60 milliliters
⅓ cup = 80 milliliters
½ cup = 120 milliliters
⅔ cup = 160 milliliters
¾ cup = 180 milliliters
1 cup = 240 milliliters
1 pint (2 cups) = 480 milliliters
1 quart (4 cups) = 960 milliliters (.96 liters)

Equivalents for Dry Measurements

AMOUNT	FINE POWDER (FLOUR)	GRAIN (RICE)
1 cup	140 grams	150 grams
¾ cup	105 grams	113 grams
⅔ cup	93 grams	100 grams
½ cup	70 grams	75 grams
⅓ cup	47 grams	50 grams
¼ cup	35 grams	38 grams
⅛ cup	18 grams	19 grams

AMOUNT	GRANULAR (SUGAR)	SOLIDS (BUTTER)
1 cup	190 grams	200 grams
¾ cup	143 grams	150 grams
⅔ cup	125 grams	133 grams
½ cup	95 grams	100 grams
⅓ cup	63 grams	67 grams
¼ cup	48 grams	50 grams
⅛ cup	24 grams	15 grams

Oven Temperatures

	FAHRENHEIT	CELSIUS	GAS MARK
Freeze water	32°F	0°C	
Room temperature	68°F	20°C	
Boil water	212°F	100°C	
Bake	325°F	160°C	3
	350°F	180°C	4
	375°F	190°C	5
	400°F	200°C	6
	425°F	220°C	7
	450°F	230°C	8

Equivalents for Weight

1 ounce = 30 grams
4 ounces = 120 grams
8 ounces = 240 grams
12 ounces = ¾ pound = 360 grams
16 ounces = 1 pound = 480 grams

Equivalents for Length

1 inch = 2.5 centimeters
6 inches = ½ foot = 15 centimeters
12 inches = 1 foot = 30 centimeters
36 inches = 3 feet = 1 yard = 90 centimeters
40 inches = 100 centimeters = 1 meter

INDEX